MULTILINGUAL ENVIRONMENTAL COMMUNICATIONS

Based on real-life case studies, this book provides an empirical study of the linguistic accessibility of environmental information for people from diverse language, cultural, and educational backgrounds. It deploys well-established statistical and machine learning models to evaluate the key linguistic features of environmental information dissemination, to both English- and non-English-speaking readers, on topics such as environmental health risk and natural disaster preparedness. Using Japanese, Swahili, Tigrinya, Zulu, and Somali languages as illustrations, this book shows how English-speaking professionals can significantly improve the cross-lingual translatability of community-oriented environmental information by using machine learning. It can be used as a latest research reference for readers from different disciplinary backgrounds interested in how to design linguistically accessible environmental information to increase its social and community impact. It can also be used as a practical guide to community-oriented environmental information design.

MENG JI is Professor at the School of Languages and Cultures, The University of Sydney, Australia. For two decades, her work has pioneered translation research innovation, through developing interdisciplinary research methods and models.

MICHAEL OAKES is Visiting Assistant Professor at the University of Birmingham, UK. His research interests are in Statistics for Corpus Linguistics, Authorship Attribution and Empirical Translation Studies.

CAMBRIDGE STUDIES IN LANGUAGE PRACTICES AND SOCIAL DEVELOPMENT

Series editors

Meng Ji, *University of Sydney*
Georges Bastin, *University of Montreal*

Language practices play an instrumental role in the development of societies, cultures, and traditions. The Cambridge Studies in Language Practices and Social Development series publishes pioneering and innovative research from around the world which explores the nexuses between the use of language by communities, individuals, specialists, technology, the media, policy makers, and the wider social, economic, cultural, and environmental changes that have shaped and continue to shape our contemporary world. This series will discuss some of the key topics in language studies which will have important implications for a sustainable and equitable society, including: the accessibility of health and environmental information for communities and individuals from disadvantaged backgrounds; the impact of generative artificial intelligence on language education; the language identity of diaspora and ethnic minorities; and the intersectionality of disability and diversity in multicultural and multilingual societies. Titles in the series are authored by established and up-and-coming scholars from diverse disciplinary backgrounds who share a common interest and passion to leverage language to bring about positive social changes for a sustainable and equitable future for all.

A full list of titles in the series can be found at www.cambridge.org/LPSD.

MULTILINGUAL ENVIRONMENTAL COMMUNICATIONS

Language Accessibility Matters

MENG JI
University of Sydney

MICHAEL OAKES
University of Birmingham

CAMBRIDGE
UNIVERSITY PRESS

CAMBRIDGE
UNIVERSITY PRESS

Shaftesbury Road, Cambridge CB2 8EA, United Kingdom

One Liberty Plaza, 20th Floor, New York, NY 10006, USA

477 Williamstown Road, Port Melbourne, VIC 3207, Australia

314–321, 3rd Floor, Plot 3, Splendor Forum, Jasola District Centre,
New Delhi – 110025, India

103 Penang Road, #05–06/07, Visioncrest Commercial, Singapore 238467

Cambridge University Press is part of Cambridge University Press & Assessment,
a department of the University of Cambridge.

We share the University's mission to contribute to society through the pursuit of education, learning and research at the highest international levels of excellence.

www.cambridge.org
Information on this title: www.cambridge.org/9781316512463

DOI: 10.1017/9781009067386

When citing this work, please include a reference to the DOI 10.1017/9781009067386

First published 2025

A catalogue record for this publication is available from the British Library

Library of Congress Cataloging-in-Publication Data
NAMES: Ji, Meng (Professor of translation studies), author. | Oakes, Michael P., author.
TITLE: Multilingual environmental communications : language accessibility matters / Meng Ji, Michael Oakes.
DESCRIPTION: Cambridge, United Kingdom ; New York, NY : Cambridge University Press, 2025. | Series: Cambridge studies in language practices and social development | Includes bibliographical references and index.
IDENTIFIERS: LCCN 2024036788 (print) | LCCN 2024036789 (ebook) | ISBN 9781316512463 (hardback) | ISBN 9781009066013 (paperback) | ISBN 9781009067386 (ebook)
SUBJECTS: LCSH: Environmental health – Translating. | Health risk communication. | Readability (Literary style) | Machine translating. | LCGFT: Case studies.
CLASSIFICATION: LCC RA423.2 .J5 2025 (print) | LCC RA423.2 (ebook) | DDC 613/.1014–dc23/eng/20241029
LC record available at https://lccn.loc.gov/2024036788
LC ebook record available at https://lccn.loc.gov/2024036789

ISBN 978-1-316-51246-3 Hardback

Contents

Figures

Tables

CHAPTER 1

Previous Research on Language Readability

1.1 Introduction

Martinc, Pollak, & Robnik-Šikonja (2021) state 'Readability is concerned with the relation between a given text and the cognitive load of a reader to comprehend it.' It thus depends on many factors: lexical, syntactic, cohesive and background knowledge. Some of these can be measured directly, particularly lexical features, but less so for syntax and cohesion, and background knowledge is very difficult to objectively measure. Thus, traditional readability measures consider lexical features such as word length, sentence length, word difficulty, n-grams (sequences of a number of consecutive words or characters), the type-token ratio (TTR) which is number of unique words in the text divided by the total number of words, and parts-of-speech (POS) related, such as number of nouns, or ratio of function words to content words. In this chapter we will follow the classification of Martinc et al. (2021) by first considering lexical features for use in readability measures, then go on to the next stage and look at syntactic and discourse properties of texts, even though they tend not to work as well as lexical or semantic properties of texts. Syntactic features include such things as average parse tree height, or the average length of a syntactic unit. Working with a French language corpus, Todirascu, François, Bernhard, Gala, & Ligozat (2016) studied sixty-five discourse features such as lexical chains (words in a text which are related by hyponymy or hypernymy) but found that they contributed little to the predictive power of text readability classifiers when compared with traditional formulas.

The third stage is machine learning, where readability is regarded as a classification (is a text of high or low readability), regression (how does readability vary as the value of a linguistic feature varies) or a ranking task – is one text more readable than another. Machine learning produces better prediction than traditional approaches, but holds a disadvantage in that we need a training set of texts each characterised by a group of linguistic features and a human-assigned category label. Related to this, another problem is that the feature sets might work well on one corpus of texts, but not another. Other approaches they consider include language modelling, and recent work on deep learning.

1.2 Traditional Readability Measures

Martinc et al. (2021) list a number of widely used traditional readability measures:

Gunning Fog Index (GFI) (Gunning, 1952):

$$GFI = 0.4\left(\frac{totalWords}{totalSentences} + 100\frac{longWords}{totalSentences}\right)$$

Long words are those which have more than seven characters. GFI is the number of years of formal schooling required to understand the text, so a higher GFI means lower readability.

Flesch Reading Ease (Kincaid, Fishburne, Rogers, & Chissom, 1975), where a higher value of FRE means the text is more readable:

$$FRE = 206.835 - 1.05\left(\frac{totalWords}{totalSentences}\right) - 84.6\left(\frac{totalSyllables}{totalWords}\right)$$

The Flesch-Kincaid Grade Level is an adaptation of the FRE to give the required grade level:

$$FKGL = 0.39\left(\frac{totalWords}{totalSentences}\right) + 11.8\left(\frac{totalSyllables}{totalWords}\right)$$

The Automated Readability Index (ARI) (Smith & Senter, 1967) also gives a value for the GFI.

$$ARI = 4.71\left(\frac{totalCharacters}{totalWords}\right) + 0.5\left(\frac{totalWords}{totalSentences}\right)$$

The Dale-Chall readability formula (DCRF) (1949) uses a list of 3,000 words that a typical fourth-grade student could easily understand. Other words are 'difficult.' If the list of 3,000 words is not available, we can assume that words with more than seven characters are difficult.

$$DCRF = 0.1579\left(\frac{difficultWords}{totalWords}\right) + 0.0496\left(\frac{totalWords}{totalSentences}\right)$$

The Simple Measure of Gobbledygook (SMOG) measure, originally used for the health domain, gives the grade level (McLaughlin, 1969). Polysyllables are words with three or more syllables:

$$SMOG = 1.0430\sqrt{numberOfPolysyllables\frac{30}{TotalSentences}} + 3.1291$$

1.2.1 *Derivation of Early Readability Formulas*

A number of costly mistakes have been made involving US Navy personnel, due to the training materials which had to be read in order to do a job, being written at a level of difficultly much above the reading ability of the man assigned to do the task (Kincaid et al., 1975). Training manuals which were more difficult to read resulted in more errors. There is thus a significant need in the armed services for readability measures which ensure that the reading levels of training manuals are not greater than the reading ability (denoted by the grade level) of the people who need to learn from them. Reducing the reading difficulty of texts is less expensive and time consuming than offering remedial reading instruction to staff or selecting only those personnel with high reading ability. Most reading formulas have been developed using members of the general population but had hitherto not been developed for US Navy personnel in particular. It was felt that the high number of technical terms in the Navy training manuals would cause readability measures to return grade levels which were too high. This problem was originally addressed by Caylor, Swift, Fox & Ford (1972), who derived the FORCAST formula for the Army from readability experiments specifically with Army personnel, but this formula includes a count of the one-syllable words in a passage, which at that time (and even today) was difficult to automate.

The grade level (in the US education system) required to read each sample text when deriving a readability formula was assigned if 50 per cent of the subjects reading that text scored 35 per cent or better on a Cloze test. In this Cloze test, every fifth word was left blank, and the reader's task was to fill each blank in. Flesch (1948) estimated that a success rate of 35 per cent to 40 per cent on the Cloze test was equivalent to a score of 75 per cent in a multiple choice test, so this criterion could also be used to determine whether the text was readable by people at a certain grade level. The Cloze test is preferable, as the questions are prepared by a more objective procedure. An example of the Cloze test is as follows:

> Preheating involves raising the temperature of the base metal or a section of the base metal above the ambient temperature before welding. (first line of welding instructions, underlined words omitted)

Once the passages were graded, the multiple regression technique described in Chapter 2 was used to derive a new formula specifically for Army use. Similarly, FORCAST, the Flesch Reading Ease formula and another readability measure called the ARI Fog Count can all be made specific to a given subset of the population by recalculating new regression formulas. The ARI test needs a modified typewriter, but the other two can be calculated without specialised equipment. Klare (1963) automated FORCAST and the Flesch measure with computer programmes which can count the number of syllables in a text, said to be accurate to ± 1 per cent. Since all three measures give their results in terms of the grade level required to understand the texts, they should in theory be interchangeable.

As long ago as 1934, Dale and Tyler wanted to determine the readability of health education articles collected from books, newspapers and magazines on the subject of health education. In doing so, they piloted much of the original methodology for deriving readability formulas for a given topic area and subset of the population, in this case adults with poor reading ability. They found twenty-nine characteristics of texts thought to influence readability and correlated these with comprehension using Pearson's product-moment regression coefficient. Ten of these correlated significantly with comprehension and three were retained for inclusion in a readability formula.

Gray and Leary (1935) found eighty-two factors related to readability by studying existing reading materials, and recommendations of adult students, teachers and academics. Eighteen of these factors would be difficult to use in readability formulas, such as 'image-bearing words' which 'defy objective measurement.' Others were discarded because they were rare in the sampled texts. Twenty factors were retained because they correlated significantly (with a correlation coefficient $r > .27$) with the comprehension test scores of adult readers.

Smith and Kincaid (1970) warn that readability measures are estimates of difficulty and should not be taken as indicators of writing quality. Deliberately trying to write according to the formula criteria, such as shortening sentence or word length, does not necessarily improve writing, and may even degrade it.

Preferred early measures are Dale-Chall for its predictive power, followed by the Flesch formula which has the advantage of not needing a special word list. Custom formulas or special adaptations of existing formulas are needed for special populations, such as children.

1.3 Machine Learning

There is a section on machine learning in general in Chapter 2. For now, let us describe it briefly as follows: Let us take a machine learning classifier as a black box, where we know what goes in and what comes out, but for now ignore the mechanism by which the input is transformed into the output. There are two stages to its operation. First, in the training phase, we submit examples of texts and with each, a readability score assigned by a human assessor. At the end of this phase, the machine learning classifier will have learned to distinguish between texts with different degrees of readability. The texts are characterised by a typically large set of linguistic features. Second, in the testing phase, new documents, also characterised by a set of their linguistic features, are shown to the classifier, which will now be able to automatically classify them.

Curtotti, McCreath, Bruce, Frug, Weibel, & Ceynowa (2015) were interested in the accessibility of legal language to e general public. Their corpus was built from the U.S. Code of Federal Regulations, which provided both training and testing data. Gold standard (definitive) labelling of the texts was achieved by crowdsourcing, where the texts are labelled online by a large number of paid volunteers. The texts were characterised by linguistic features extracted using the Stanford dependency grammar parser and the Stanford context free parser. This enabled them to predict the readability of legal texts with high accuracy.

Kanungo and Orr (2009) looked at the readability of web page summaries or 'gists', which are frequently given to accompany the 'hit lists' provided as output by commercial search engines. It would be time consuming and expensive to provide readability assessments manually, and this would not be possible to do in real-time when people were actually using the search engines. However, once the machine learning classifier had been trained, it was possible to assign a readability score to each web page gist automatically. Once again, the machine learning classifier outperformed traditional readability measures. The learning algorithm, called a 'gradient-boosted decision tree', enabled the later extraction of linguistic features thought to influence readability.

Kotani, Yoshimi, & Isahara (2011)'s work focused on the readability of English texts to Japanese learners of the language. The subjects were instructed to read each text carefully, until they were able to answer a comprehension question. So that they did not feel under pressure and rush the task, they were not told that the time taken to answer the questions was being recorded. They used regression to estimate text readability based on comprehension rate and lexical, syntactic and discourse factors, such as the number of pronouns, as this requires the discourse task of identifying their referents.

In a highly novel departure from characterising texts by their linguistic features, Victoria Yaneva (2016) collected eye-tracking data while subjects were reading web pages, and used the patterns in the gaze track to characterise the texts. She was interested in evaluating and improving web site access for people with an autistic spectrum disorder (ASD), and the collected eye movement traces were stored in the ASD corpus. For the training phase, sets of traces obtained from subjects reading texts pre-classified as easy, medium or difficult were presented to the classifier. Then in the test phase, reading difficulty could be estimated from the gaze tracks alone. From these experiments, Yaneva was able to compile a set of guidelines for improving text readability.

Buse and Weimer (2008) studied the readability not of text, but of computer code. They expected beforehand that this would depend on such things as indentation, choice of identifier names and the presence or otherwise of natural language comments to explain the following code sections. They used the Weka machine learning toolbox, which enables the operation of many different machine learning classifiers. They found that the main features degrading code readability were the average number of identifiers per line, the average line length, the average number of brackets ('{' or '(') per line, and the maximum line length. A few features were found to improve the readability of computer code: the average number of blank lines, the average length of comments, and surprisingly, there was a small beneficial effect of average number per line of the arithmetic operation symbols '+', '*', '%', '/' and '-'.

1.3.1 *Training Corpora for Machine Learning Approaches*

An early example of a supervised learning approach (Schwarm & Ostendorf, 2005) used a Support Vector Machine (SVM) trained on a corpus built from the now defunct children's magazine *Weekly Reader*, which contains articles grouped according to four reader age classes. More recent work using this corpus is described by Petersen and Ostendorf (2009). The OneStopEnglish corpus has three readability classes (Vajjala & Lučić, 2018). Vajjala and Lučić used 155 linguistic features and the Sequential Minimal Optimization (SMO) classifier. The WeeBit corpus has texts divided into five readability classes (see Vajjala & Meurers, 2012) who used an early neural network approach called a multilayer perceptron. The WeeBit corpus annotations correspond to the age groups 7–8, 8–9, 9–10, 10–14, and 14–16 years. The three younger groups consist of articles from Weekly Reader, while the texts for the older groups come from the BBC-Bitesize website. The original corpus was built by Vajjala and Meurers (2012), but a version was later cleaned and used by Xia, Kochmar, and Briscoe (2016). The final corpus consisted of 3,000 documents, with 600 per age category. It is not a parallel corpus, so the texts at each level are unrelated to each other.

The Newsela Corpus (Xu, Callison-Burch, & Napoles, 2015) texts come from the Newsela company that produces reading materials for primary and secondary school pupils. It is a parallel corpus (showing which sentences of one side correspond with which sentence or sentences of the other side) of original and simplified texts at each grade from the second to the eleventh. There is not always the same number of texts for each grade, but there are 10,786 texts overall, produced from 1,911 originals. Other corpora used for training readability classifiers are Britannica (with adult and elementary versions of the same texts), and Convolutional Neural Networks (CNN) (with adult and abridged versions of the texts). The Common European Framework of Reference for Languages (CEFR) corpus is small, but has five levels of graded texts for English learners. The OneStopEnglish corpus (Vajjala & Lučić, 2018) consists of aligned text at three reading levels, and was created for English as a Second Language (ESL) learners. The texts originally came from *The Guardian* newspaper, and were simplified in two stages. It consists of 189 texts each at three levels. Martinc et al. (2021) used some of these corpora, and also used a corpus of Slovenian school books.

1.4 Language Model Features

An example of a language model is a Markov model. In a Markov model, the likelihood of a word or Part of Speech (POS) being seen depends on its inherent likelihood and the identity of a number of previous symbols. To take an example at the character level, the likelihood of encountering the letter 'u' at a certain position in the text depends on how common the letter 'u' is in general and the previous characters. If the immediately preceding character is 'q', then the next character is highly likely to be a 'u.' A language model trained on one corpus is evaluated according to how well it predicts a separate test sequence of words, using the measure of perplexity (PPL).

$$PPL = 2^{-\frac{1}{N}\sum_{i=1}^{N} log_2 m(w_i)}$$

Where $m(w_i)$ is the probability assigned to word w_i by the language model m, and N is the length of the sequence. The lower the perplexity score, the better the language model predicts the words in a new document. Perplexity scores can be used as features in a classifier – see Xia et al., 2016.

One advantage of a language model trained on English is that it can easily be retrained (given a new probabilistic dictionary, which is a long list of words and their probabilities) to work in French as well as English (Collins-Thompson & Callan, 2004). While the Type-Token Ratio (TTR) performed better on commercially available articles with human readability ratings, this model worked best for web pages and very short texts of less than ten words. This was the result they hoped for, since they were interested in producing a search engine which returned web pages of a suitable readability level as well as being on a suitable topic.

The Flesch-Kincaid formula assumes that the text is at least 100 words long and uses clear-cut sentences, neither of which are guaranteed for web pages.

Traditional models use just two or three variables – statistical language models can use a very large number.

A number of previous readability measures use vocabulary lists, such as the Dale-Chall (1949) formula which uses a vocabulary of 3,000 words which are easy to understand. These word lists act as simple language models, since each word in the list is implicitly given a score of 1 (for present) and each word not in the list a score of 0 (for absent). The method of Collins-Thompson and Callan (2004) uses more sophisticated language models since each word in the model is given a probability score, which is the number of times it occurs in the training corpus divided by the total number of words in the training corpus. They are said to be 1-gram models, since they consider only the frequency of single words, not the likelihood of them occurring in a particular word sequence, which would require 2-gram or 3-gram models. In early experiments they found that the more abstract a word, the more likely it is to be used at higher readability levels. This opens up the possibility of distinguishing between possible grade levels of a text by using the relative frequencies of the words in them.

They built a corpus of 550 web pages which were specifically written for readers at various grade levels. In these texts, concrete words such as 'red' were found most often at low grade levels, most typically 2; more abstract words such as 'perimeter' found peak usage at grade level 6, falling off at either side; 'determine' was most used at grade level 11. These results show that distinguishing readability by grade according to the abstractness of the vocabulary is feasible. If $L(G_i|T)$ is the likelihood of text T having the readability of Grade i (where for example G5 is Grade 5), C(w) is the count of word w in text T, and $P(w|G_i)$ is the probability value for word w in the training corpus for G_i, then

$$L(G_i|T) = \sum_{w \in T} C(w) log P(w|G_i)$$

Thus for each grade level we work out the likelihood of our text having that degree of readability (so we work out the formula twelve times, one for each grade level). To do this for one grade level, we find for every word the number of times it occurs in the text and multiply it by the logarithm (function on a standard calculator) of the word's probability value in the training corpus of the language model. These products are then all added together. The language model with the highest likelihood is chosen as the one corresponding to the most probable reading level of the text.

The language models are smoothed, so that words which are nonexistent or very rare in the training corpora have their probabilities increased by a small amount, so 'nothing is impossible.' Language models are often created from the Wikipedia dump.

1.5 Deep Learning

Machine Learning techniques like SVM tend to be highly accurate. A subfield of machine learning is called deep learning. Deep learning models have the additional advantage of not requiring prior feature extraction: the inputs tend to be raw text, and in the case of readability measurements, the outputs tend to be either reading level categories or real-valued readability scores. Deep learning has the disadvantages that they can take a long time to train, the programmer is responsible for setting the fine-tuning parameters, and they may be hard to debug. Deep learning stems from the older paradigm of neural networks, which are inspired by the biological network of the human brain. In a neural network, a set of nodes, which roughly represent brain cells, is arranged in layers, where the inputs (such as a set of linguistic features) are presented to the input layer, and the output (in our case) could be one node representing a readability value. Between the input layer and the output layer is the hidden layer of nodes. Each node has a cell body and a nerve called an axon, connecting it to other nodes. When a cell receives sufficient input from other nodes or the input features, it can 'fire' and stimulate nodes in the next layer. It is the number of layers which distinguish deep learning from the older neural networks. Deep Learning must have more than three layers, which has become possible relatively recently as modern computers have greater processing power than before. However, in this chapter, we use the terms deep learning and neural network interchangeably. Deep learning may be supervised (requiring a training set of examples previously categorised by human experts) or unsupervised (where it learns to categorise data without any human intervention). Commonly-used examples of deep learning, which we will cover briefly in this section are Convolutional Neural Networks (CNN), Recurrent Neural Networks (RNN) and Long Short Term Memory (LSTM). Both CNN and LSTM have been widely and successfully used in the field of Natural Language Processing. It is thought that CNN is good at capturing local features of language, while LSTM is good at processing sequence data (like words in a sentence) and capturing long-distance dependencies (such as anaphora resolution) (Jian, Xiang, & Le, 2022). Neural models outperform n-gram language models because they look at a wider context. There is a general maximum of 5 for n-grams due to data sparseness (Martinc et al., 2021).

Readability measures are relevant to tasks like text simplification and for teachers selecting materials at the right level for their students (Nadeem & Ostendorf, 2018). Traditional methods using linguistic features as inputs have the advantage of being easy to interpret. However, they have the disadvantages of not working well with short texts, and not generalising well to new domains, such as from literature to science. Sheehan, Flor, & Naplitano (2013) showed that traditional readability measures tend to underestimate the reading level of literary texts, while they tend to over-estimate the reading level of 'informational' texts, such as those in history, science and mathematics. In fact, they recommend a two-stage process, with genre identification as a precursor of readability measurement. Nadeem and Ostendorf's (2018) neural approach succeeded in overcoming both problems. They used a type of neural network called a RNN which requires no set of linguistic features as input, but instead is able to generalise a likely reading level from the raw text input.

Recurrent Neural Networks have been used in a number of text representation tasks, most notably the Word2Vec architecture of Mikolov, Karafiát, Burget, Černocký, & Khudanpur (2010), which represents a word in the input text by a vector (list) of the collocational strengths of other words found in its context. So-called attention mechanisms can be shown to improve text processing tasks such as classification and machine translation (Nadeem & Ostendorf, 2018). These enable the neural network to focus on those parts of the input text which most contribute to the decision on grade level.

Uses of readability measurement include book recommendation or classification, web page summarisation for use with search engines, and (the focus of this book) accessibility in the health domain (Azpiazu & Pera, 2019).

Although neural networks can work using only raw text for input, circumventing the task of linguistic feature extraction, the system described here (called Vec2Read) also accepts part-of-speech and morphological information, such as person and tense. Azpiazu and Pera (2019) present a multiattentive recurrent neural network architecture for multilingual readability assessment. A RNN is a development of a traditional neural network in which each layer accepts not only inputs from the previous layer, but also an input from the immediately adjacent node in the same layer, representing information from previous words in the text (as words in a text are dependent on each other). RNNs have the problem that they are difficult to train, but Azpiazu and Pera (2019) overcame this difficulty by using an extension of the RNN called a LSTM which enables its neurons to either remember or forget certain information. They also used other types of neural networks.

In recent years, neural networks have outperformed approaches based on linguistically motivated features. Deutsch, Jasbi, & Scheiber (2020) tried adding linguistic information to the output of a neural network, but found that this did not lead to significant improvement. They hypothesised that their deep learning neural networks had already learnt all the linguistic information that could be gleaned from the raw text, both surface level and deeper factors, and thus the addition of more linguistic information was superfluous. They combined the deep learning model outputs with the traditional linguistic features by using them all as features for SVMs, a traditional machine learning architecture. A similar approach is taken in Chapter 3 of this book, where outputs of traditional readability measures are used as inputs for an SVM, alongside raw linguistic features.

Yancey, Pintard, & François (2021) present the first readability model for French as a Foreign Language (FFL) based on a deep-learning model, which outperformed the state-of-the-art. As well as features generated by the outputs of deep learning, they used cognitive features. Both types of features were incorporated into an SVM. The cognitive features included the proportion of abstract and concrete words, where more concrete words tend to be more easily recognised. They also used the Orthographic Levenshtein Distance 20 (OLD20), where Levenshtein Distance is the number of edits (insertions, deletions or substitutions) required to transform one word into another. The OLD20 version returns the average Levenshtein distance taken over the closest twenty words found in the lexicon. The rationale is that the existence of a large number of orthographic neighbours (similarly spelled words) results in interference when reading, producing lower readability. The third cognitive criterion was the average number of commonly known senses per word, as found in the large semantic network Babelnet, which if greater, tends to produce poorer readability. Their evaluation criteria were accuracy, the proportion of times that the machine assigned texts the same grade level as human assessors, adjacent accuracy which is like accuracy but also allows the classifications to differ by 1, and the Pearson product-moment correlation coefficient between the set of humanly-assigned grade scores for each text and the corresponding machine-calculated grades.

1.6 Readability Measures in Other Languages

Azpiazu and Pera (2020) state that readability formulas are rarely consistent when measuring translations of the same text. There was thus a need to develop measures of readability for texts in languages other than English. The four stages in development of such measures seem to be firstly to use a formula designed for English exactly as it is, but on other language texts; secondly to adapt these English formulas according to the quantitative characteristics of the language pair, such as relative word length; thirdly to develop formulas completely afresh for the other language; and finally there is a trend in several languages to machine learning and deep learning approaches. This chapter will concentrate on three languages for which considerable work on readability has been done, namely Italian, Swedish and French. We will also briefly describe individual case studies for German and two Indian languages.

Chapter 5 will describe in detail some work on readability in Japanese. Sung, Chang, Lin, Hsieh, & Chang (2016) used an SVM with twenty-four linguistic features to predict text readability in Chinese. Correia and Mendes (2021) describe a deep learning model for measuring the readability score of texts in European Portuguese. See Škvorc, Krek, Pollak, & Arhad Holdt (2018) for Slovenian.

1.6.1 Readability in Italian

The earliest readability index for Italian was Flesch-Vacca which was derived from the Flesch index for English. The Flesch index version they used was F = 206.385 – (84.6 × S) – (1.015 × P) where F is readability, S is the average number of syllables per paragraph, and P is the average number of words per sentence. Roberto Vacca and Valerio Franchina proposed the following adaptation for the Italian language:

$$\mathrm{F} = 206 - (0.65 \times \mathrm{S}) - \mathrm{P}$$

Instead of counting the length of words and sentences in syllables, Gulpease (Lucisano & Piemontese, 1988) uses the number of letters, giving a simpler calculation, where counts for sentences, letters and words are those for the entire document.

$$F = 89 + \frac{300 \times numberofsentences - 10 \times numberofletters}{numberofwords}$$

F should be in the range 0 to 100, where 0 is the most difficult. However, it is not constrained to be in this range. For example, texts with F > 40 should be legible by students with high school diplomas, and texts with F > 60 can normally be read by students with a middle school diploma, and texts with F > 80 can normally be read by students with a primary school diploma.

The system of Tonelli, Tran Manh, & Pianta (2012) accepts documents in the Italian language, and outputs a set of readability metrics inspired by Coh-Metrix (Graesser et al., 2004; http://cohmetrix.memphis.edu), which is a package able to calculate about sixty readability-related aspects of an input text. Coh-Metrix takes advantage of recent work in psycholinguistics and natural language processing such as dependency and constituency parsers, and anaphora resolution. The system also displays how each measure compares with three levels of Italian education – elementary, middle and high school. The aim of the research by Tonelli et al. (2012) was to improve web content readability.

Three Coh-Metrix indices were derived by collecting texts written by three groups of people: children in elementary schools, children aged 11–13 in middle schools, and teenagers in high schools. A similar approach had been advocated by Crossley, Allan, & McNamara (2011), who used original and manually simplified texts. The linguistic features measured by Coh-Metrix are in five main classes: First, general word and text information such as syllables per word and the TTR. If these are high, it seems likely that the sentence would be more difficult to process cognitively and hence more difficult to read. Similarly sentences with greater syntactic complexity, such as those with a greater number of embedded constituents will be more difficult to read. Third, referential and semantic indexes. For example, if a sentence is not cohesive with respect to adjacent sentences it is more difficult to process. Fourth, indices for the complexity of a mental model evoked by a document (see Dijk & Kintsch, 1983) and lastly existing measures such as Flesch Reading Ease. The online demonstration of CohMetrix shows about sixty such measures. Syllables were computed using the Perl module Lingua::IT::Hyphenate: see http://search.cpan.org/~acalpini/Lingua-IT-Hyphenate.

The Italian adaptation of Coh-Metrix is called Coease. Here features 1 – 6 are basic features of the text such as number of words or syllables. Features 7 to 10 consider the familiarity of words using a frequency list from the whole of the Italian Wikipedia at that time – Low frequency words are less familiar. Index 8, the logarithm of the raw frequency of content words was used, as this psycholinguistic measure relates to reading time (Haberlandt & Graesser, 1985). Content words can be estimated as those with parts-of-speech verb, adjective and noun. Indices 11–12 measure the abstractness of nouns. One way of doing this would be to look at the level of the word in the MultiWordNet hierarchy (Pianta, Bentivogli, & Girardi, 2002). Indices 20–29 capture cohesion of sentences by looking at connectives. Indices 30–31 relate to the syntactic similarity of sentences – high syntactic variability in a text being easier to understand.

The purpose of assessing readability in the READ-IT project was to evaluate text simplification for newspapers. Potential beneficiaries were people with low literacy skills, both native speakers and learners of Italian. Health-related information was another crucial domain where it was desired to make the information available to a large and heterogeneous reader group. READ-IT used a SVM. Different linguistic features came into play according to whether the readers were L1 or L2 learners. Four levels of features proposed by the READ-IT project corresponded with the NLP tools required to calculate them.

First, the raw text features typically used in traditional metrics such as word and sentence length. The tools needed to extract them included tokenisers. Second, they used lexical features such as those extracted by lemmatisers, including the lemmas in the Basic Italian Vocabulary by De Mauro (2000). This contains a list of 7,000 frequently used Italian words. They also used the TTR. Here there is a requirement for text samples of equal length, as TTR decreases as texts get larger and fewer new words are introduced. Morpho-syntactic features were extracted by such tools as part-of-speech (PoS) tagging, such as the Language Modelling probability of PoS unigrams, and lexical density, which is the ratio of content words to all tokens in the text. Verbal mood was a feature specifically for Italian. Syntactic tools were extracted by dependency parsers, which allowed the calculation of such measures as parse-tree depth features (including whole-tree parse tree depth), and the longest path from the root of the dependency tree to some leaf, and the length of dependency links (equal to the number of words occurring between the syntactic head and the dependent, or phrase length). The corpus used to extract the linguistic features was La Repubblica, a highly readable newspaper. The morpho-syntactic features were the most reliable, producing 98 per cent accuracy.

1.6.2 *Readability in Swedish*

The most widely used metric in Swedish is LIX, the Läsbarhets (Readability) Index of Björnsson (1968). Based on the Flesch score, it can be applied to texts written in any language, since it depends only on word length, sentence length and the number of 'difficult' words, namely those of more than six characters. LIX = 100(B/W) + (W/S) = per cent of long words plus average words per sentence. A score of 20 would suggest a simple text and one of 60 a highly complex text.

The OVIX (Ordsvariationsindex or Word Variation Index) and the Nominal Ratio (Hultman & Westman, 1977) were developed later as they correlated better with features taken from higher linguistic levels, which have been made possible to count by the advent of text analysis tools such as grammars and parsers. The OVIX formula is given by King (2019).

$$OVIX = \frac{\log(\textit{total number of words})}{\log\left(2 - \frac{\log(\textit{number of unique words})}{\log(\textit{total number of words})}\right)}$$

King gives these six easy steps for working out this formula:

1. Find the logarithm of the total number of words (tokens) in the sample.

2. Find the logarithm of the number of unique words (types) in the sample.
3. Divide the result of step 2 by the result of step 1.
4. Subtract the result of step 3 from 2 (the number 2, not the result of step 2)
5. Find the natural logarithm of the result of step 4.
6. Divide the result of step 1 by the result of step 5.

Falkenjack, Heimann Mühlenbock, & Jönsson (2013) created a training corpus made up of simplified texts, called the LäsBarT corpus, and five corpora of non-simplified texts in the domains of general news, popular science, professional news, government text and fiction. This solved the problem of text annotation, as according to the origin of the texts they could automatically be labelled as 'easy-to-read' or 'not-easy-to-read.' The machine learning algorithm they used was SVM (used successfully in other readability experiments, such as Feng et al. (2010), who used the Waikato Environment for Knowledge Analysis (Weka) package (Garner, 1995)). As was done with the READ-IT system, a set of candidate features found in the literature was subdivided into shallow (requiring tokenisation), lexical (requiring lemmatisation), morpho-syntactic (needing part-of-speech tagging), and syntactic (requiring parsing). Best accuracy when using single feature models was obtained for unigram dependency type (the unigram probabilities for the sixty-three dependency types per token) closely followed by the unigram part-of-speech type per token, where each part-of-speech ratio acted as an individual attribute.

In this section we contrast traditional readability measures with an approach which combines automated linguistic analysis with machine learning. Falkenjack et al. (2013) follow a similar approach, and look at the extent to which linguistic features proposed for other languages, especially English, are suitable for determining readability in Swedish. They found that the best performing features were sequences of part-of-speech tags and syntactic dependency type.

Reasons for measuring readability in text include giving teachers a means of assessing a student's reading ability, and advising general readers that they might consider looking for easier texts on the same topic – and readability measures would help them find such texts. In this chapter we regard readability as meaning easy-to-read, although Dale and Chall (1949), who developed one of the earliest readability formulas, define readability also as a function of how well the readers understand the text, whether they can read it at a comfortable speed, and whether they find the text interesting.

Pilán et al. (2014) studied the readability of sentences understandable to second language learners of Swedish. Most previous studies have concentrated on L1 readers. Their rule-based approach slightly outperformed the combined machine learning rule-based model. It is useful to check the readability of sentences to make sure they are suitable for automatic grading exercises. To help select linguistic indicators, they used suggestions made in previous machine learning-based readability research, aspects of Good Dictionary Examples (GDEX) (Kilgariff et al., 2008) and second language learning syllabuses. Machine Learning was able to distinguish sentences suitable for intermediate learning ('within the B1 level') from those which could be used for advanced learners 'above the B1 level.'

Traditional readability measures for Swedish include the Läsbarhets index and the Nominal Ratio. Pilán et al.'s (2014) paper is concerned with sentence-level readability as opposed to full-text readability, as they were interested in selecting appropriate vocabulary example sentences. Traditional readability measures have not been found to work so well for very short texts (Kilgariff et al., 2008). GDEX is a sentence-ranking system, which credits sentences according to such things as length, the inclusion of simple vocabulary items and the lack of anaphoric pronouns. This study used the Korp corpus, where the words are mostly POS-tagged, syntactic dependency relations, lemmas and sense identifiers. They also used frequency-based word lists, one based on the Swedish Wikipedia, and the CEFR corpus, a collection of L2 Swedish course-book texts. All of the Korp corpus was B1, while CEFR consisted of some B1 and some B2 texts.

The features used were traditional readability measures, easy-to-compute shallow features such as sentence length including punctuation and mean number of characters per token. Syntactic features were used such as the ratio of a morphosyntactic category such as adverbs to the number of content words in a sentence. Lexico-morphological features such as TTR (vocabulary diversity) were also used, the rarity of words using the Wikipedia word list being found to work best. Semantic features, such as does a word have more than one meaning, as determined by the meaning (sense) codes in an automatic tagger? were used as well. It is possible to find the most important features 'weightings' after the event in machine learning – the best was percentage of words above the B1 level. Classification accuracy for the SVM was about 71 per cent, comparable to the value obtained by previous authors for similar tasks.

Larsson (2006) presented a SVM classifier for Swedish readability levels. The corpus consisted of quality newspaper texts as the more difficult-to-read, high-school texts to represent medium level readability, and easy-to-read tabloid newspapers.

1.6.3 Readability in French

A review of early readability measures for French is given by Benoit (1986). The earliest readability measures for French were adaptations of the American Flesch score. Kandel and Moles (1958) produced a light modification of the English language Flesch formula, taking into account that on average, words in French are a little bit longer than English words. More widely used is the adaptation of Landsheere (1963): Facilité = 206.835 – (X + Y). In general, there is a correlation between sentence or word length and difficulty. Thus X is a syntactic variable, namely the average length of sentences expressed in words. This number is multiplied by a coefficient of 1.015. Y is the lexical variable, the number of syllables per 100 words, multiplied by 0.85. This formula results in a value between 0 (practically illegible) and 100 (easy for any literate person). In deriving this formula, the corpus consisted of excerpts from textbooks with reading difficulty defined in the Common European Framework of Reference for Languages (CEFR) (Council of Europe, 2001) at six levels: A1 Breakthrough; A2 Waystage; B1 Threshold; B2 Vantage; C1 Effective Operational Proficiency and C2 Mastery (François and Fairon, 2012).

Landsheere's student, Georges Henry (1975), produced the first original set of formulas for French. The most complicated one has 26 parameters and requires computer calculation. The simplest, called the manual method, only three variables: syntax (number of words per phrase as in the Dale-Chall formula), and vocabulary not in the Gougenheim list of simple words (excluding proper nouns, and technical terms defined in the text), and dialogue and dramatisation markers such as first names, quotation marks and exclamation marks). Using two of these three variables, we may read off the Henry score from a set of curves on a graph. The curves on the graph appear one above another and correspond to the number of difficult words per hundred words (the greater the number, the lower the curve). We read off the syntactic variable on the horizontal axis, then look directly up to the relevant vocabulary curve. At the meeting point, we look directly left, and read off on the vertical axis the relevant readability score. This test was designed so that a text would ideally be in the range 35 to 45. Texts with scores over 45 would be too difficult, while those with scores less than 35 would be too easy. Three separate graphs were produced by Henry: one for first grade students, and two others for fourth and sixth grade students (Benoit, 1986).

François and Fairon (2012) used machine learning to distinguish between texts which learners of French as a foreign language (FFL) would find easy to read and which they would not. Readability features specific to FFL include the fact that Multi-Word Expressions (MWE) are known to cause difficulty for students of a language. Also variables typical of dialogue are more common in lower grade books) e.g. punctuation types. To the best of our knowledge, Uitdenbogerd's (2005) formula for the readability of French as a foreign language is the first formula to incorporate cognates, which are 'words that are recognisably similar to words with the same meaning in the person's native language'. Some books intentionally make use of cognates such as Uitdenbogerd's own comic book which used only cognates and 12 of the 20 most common words in French newspapers. To estimate readability, she took the first 100 words of each text and then continued on to the next sentence break. Cognates were manually counted: either an exact spelling, plus or minus a terminal 'e', or a syllabic word with an 'obvious' common root such as 'compliqué' (complicated). If a cognate was found more than once, it was counted just once for each time it occurred. The readability FR = 10 × WpS – Cog, where WpS is the average words per sentence and Cog is the number of cognates. The work is interesting as this is a characteristic of French as a Foreign language – more basic textbooks contain more cognates. The problem is that it was developed for only one language pair, but the method would apply to any two languages which are historically related or contain a large number of borrowings.

Collins-Thompson and Callan (2004) describe a language modelling approach to predicting reading difficulty in French.

1.6.4 Readability in German

Vor der Brück and Hartrumpf produced a semantically oriented readability checker for German. They used a parser called WOCADI (Hartfumpf, 2003) which can transform a text into a semantic net, a structure where each discrete concept is described as a node, and the relations between them are described by links. The meaning of the text is captured by the use of labels on the nodes (such as the word 'today') and links (such as the relation 'temporal'). A list of characteristics of each node concept can be stored with the name of the concept. They found that a number of characteristics of the semantic net were related to readability. For example, a text is more readable if it contains more concrete and fewer abstract nouns; fewer negations; indicators concerning anaphors; number of prepositions in the sentence; and the longest path in the semantic net. This last feature is the greatest number of links which must be traversed to go from any node to any other one in the net.

1.6.5 Readability in Indian Languages

Pantula and Kuppusamy (2020) estimated grade level by measuring the readability of web pages in Indian languages. English readability formulas are not suitable for evaluating Hindi and Bangla texts because of morphology (languages with more complex morphology produce longer sentences) and different grapheme correspondences (different numbers of characters per sound). They collected over 8,000 unique web pages, then used the Flesch-Kincaid measure to classify these web pages in two ways: First as less readable, readable and highly readable, and secondly according to minimum grade level required to understand the texts using the grade level version of the Flesch-Kincaid formula. The linguistic features of the texts, extracted using packages available with the Python programming language, included average number of words per sentence, number of sentences, and the average number of syllables per sentence. This data was used to train the classifier. More specifically, they considered 6 'readability characteristic' features (word count, average number of words per sentence, number of sentences, syllable count, average number of syllables per sentence, and number of words containing more than two syllables). Many words in a number of languages have a CVC structure, where one consonant is followed by one vowel, which in turn is followed by a consonant. If a word has a CVCVC structure, then the number of vowels is the number of syllables. This simple method, however, would not work for words such as 'make' in English. The lexical features they used included type-token ratio, rare words, defined by words containing the rare (in English) characters b, j, k, q, v, w, x, and z and lexical ambiguity. The best performing machine learning models were called Random Forest (RF) and Decision Tree Classification (DTC). They developed a browser extension to assess every uploaded web page for readability.

1.7 Conclusion

Readability formulas are important in education as teachers need to 'match learners with texts' (François & Fairon, 2012). The first step in enhancing anything is to measure it (Pantula & Kuppusamy, 2022). Readability assessment has been a key research area for the past eighty years, and still attracts researchers today. The text is not the sole determiner of readability – it also depends on the audience, where for example a text might be readable to a native speaker but not to a learner. The most common measures currently in use are Flesch-Kincaid and Dale-Chall. In the Flesch-Kincaid measure, number of syllables per word is a proxy for lexical complexity, while sentence length is a proxy for syntactic complexity (Lucisano & Piemontese, 1988).

Traditional models were parsimonious, incorporating as few linguistic features as possible, and used linear regression to combine two or three surface features. Later models used psychological theory, measuring such things as coherence, density, and inference load. The inference load for a text differs according to the user's skill and knowledge, and depends on recovering the event chains (actions, physical states and mental states) underlying the texts (Kemper, 1983). Petersen and Ostendorf looked at the inadequacy of reading formulae to argue for machine learning approaches. Thus, the period from 2000 to 2010 saw work on readability making use of more sophisticated NLP techniques such as syntactic parsing, statistical language modelling, and machine learning. The later chapters in this book look at non-traditional uses of readability measures, such as determining the suitability of texts for machine translation. In this vein, Zwitter Vitez (2014) used readability measures as features in an authorship attribution task. Sheehan et al., 2013, look at the applicability of readability formulas across genres. Another theme of this book is the focus on one genre in particular: texts on environmental health.

Liu, Ji, Shanshan Lin, Zhao, & Lyv (2021) state that readability measures based solely on linguistic features do not take account of the reader's age, health, cultural or linguistic background. Their paper describes the use of machine learning to combine linguistic features with reader background, enabling a move away from 'one size fits all' metrics. For example, words in lists such as the Dale-Chall list which form part of some readability measures may be easier to understand by some people than others. Factors include familiarity with the health education traditions in the language of the health-related texts. Difficult-to-read health information can result in confusion and medical errors.

In the study by Liu et al. (2021), texts on the topic of infectious diseases from high-quality Australian websites were rated by individual human readers, and these individual human assessments formed the gold standard for training and testing. The features were linguistic – hence we have a combination of linguistic and human readability data. The subjects were all learners of English with no specialist medical knowledge. A variety of machine learning models were used and one neural network. Key surface linguistic features were average syllables per word (showing morphological complexity) and sentence length, both form part of Flesch and Linsear, where the Linsear Write Formula is Score = (Easy Words) + (Hard Words x 3) / Sentence Count. If the number of easy words is less than twenty, divide by 2, otherwise subtract 2 then divide by 2. The Machine Learning methods performed well. Various researchers have come to the conclusion that Machine Learning methods can improve readability estimation. The process is data-driven, requiring less manual labour and avoiding human bias (Liu et al., 2021). Current research seems to focus on deep learning methods, which show great promise.

CHAPTER 2

Statistics and Machine Learning for Textual Readability Studies

2.1 Introduction

In this chapter, we aim to give an introduction to the statistics used in the experiments described in this book. First, we will describe how to characterize data, in terms of what is the most typical value in the data set, and also in terms of how spread out the data is. We will then describe what is called the normal distribution, or the 'bell curve' characteristic of how data is spread out in many areas of science. We will describe how the shape of the normal distribution enables hypothesis testing, one example of a hypothesis being 'Is the average number of characters per sentence greater in highly readable texts than in texts with low readability?' We can still do such tests even if the data is not normally distributed, using a family of tests called 'non-parametric', and we will look in detail at one such test called the Mann-Whitney test. In the section on regression, we look at how two variables or ways of measuring data are related to each other, such as the number of unique monosyllables in a text and a score related to the readability of that text. Does one tend to increase as the other does? An extension of the Mann-Whitney test is the Kruskal-Wallis test, which allows the simultaneous comparison of three or more groups of data. This can be followed by the Dunn test, which will tell us which pairwise comparisons among the groups are statistically significant. We will use simple linear regression as an introduction to multiple regression, the technique used in the development of a number of traditional readability measures. A more sophisticated form of regression is called logistic regression, and we will describe this technique which is used in Chapters 4 to 6.

Logistic regression provides a link between traditional statistics and machine learning, as it falls into both categories. Machine Learning is a general term for a wide variety of computer classifiers, where the machine, being presented with sufficient examples of already classified data, learns to tell the difference between various classes of input, such as texts of high or low readability. Once this has been achieved, new unclassified samples can be assigned the appropriate class by the machine learner. We will concentrate on the two machine learning techniques used in Chapters 4 to 6, logistic regression and Support Vector Machines. For the sake of completeness, we will also cover an example of a recent class of machine learners, what is called neural deep learning.

2.2 Characterising the Data by 'Average' and 'Spread'

Imagine ten texts are characterised by the proportion of long (six characters or more) words in them, as follows:

```
0.222 0.227 0.357 0.286 0.343 0.150 0.200 0.250 0.250 0.250
```

This data can be input into the R programming language as shown below, where 'long' is an arbitrary name for the resulting list of data.

```
long = c(0.222, 0.227, 0.357, 0.286, 0.343, 0.150, 0.200,
0.250, 0.250, 0.250)
```

To find the 'average' proportion of long words in the texts, we can use one of three measures. The first is the mean, which is found by adding all the data together (to give a sum of 2.535), then dividing by the number of texts which is ten, to give 0.2535. The relevant R command is

```
mean(long)
```

Another measure is the median, which can be found by sorting the data from smallest to largest, such as by using

```
sort(long)
```

to give the list:

```
0.150 0.200 0.222 0.227 0.250 0.250 0.250 0.286 0.343 0.357
```

The median is the figure exactly in the middle of the list. If the list has an odd number of members, then there will be a single value in the central position. Here we have ten items, an even number, so we take the fifth and sixth (both 0.250) and take the mean of these, also 0.250. The median can be calculated using a single R command, as follows:

```
median(long)
```

The third measure is the mode. This is the value which occurs most frequently in the data set. There is no direct command for finding the mode in R, but we can use the `table` command:

```
table(long)
```

which gives the response:

```
0.15 0.2 0.222 0.227 0.25 0.286 0.343 0.357
   1   1     1     1    3     1     1     1
```

This table shows that all the values in the data set were encountered just once each, except for 0.25, which was the proportion of long words in three texts. Thus the mode is 0.25. Notice that the three measures for the 'average' for this data set are not identical.

The measure of spread which most concerns us is the standard deviation. If all the values in the data set were identical, the standard deviation would be 0, but since they are mostly different, the standard deviation will be a positive value. There is no upper limit for the standard deviation. It is given by the formula:

$$s = \frac{1}{n-1} \sum_{i=1}^{n} (x_i - \bar{x})^2$$

The summation symbol Σ means that starting with the first item, when i = 1, and finishing with the last item, when i = 10, we add together all the differences between each x value and the mean x value in turn. The standard deviation for our data for the proportion of long words in a text can be calculated stepwise using Table 2.1:

Table 2.1 *Stepwise calculation of the standard deviation*

I	x_i	$(x_i - \bar{x})$	$(x_i - \bar{x})^2$
1	0.222	−0.0315	0.00099225
2	0.227	−0.0265	0.00070225
3	0.357	0.1035	0.01071225
4	0.286	0.0325	0.00105625
5	0.343	0.0895	0.00801025
6	0.150	−0.1035	0.01071225
7	0.200	−0.0535	0.00286225
8	0.250	−0.0035	0.00001225
9	0.250	−0.0035	0.00001225
10	0.250	−0.0035	0.00001225
	$\bar{x}$= 02535		Sum = 0.0350845
			$\sqrt{\text{Sum}/(10-1)} = 0.06243619$

In the first column we write the text number, and in the second column we write the corresponding proportion of long words for that text. We then add these values and divide by the number of texts to find the mean. In the third column we find the difference between the value for each individual text and the mean. We do not add these together to find the sum, because we know that some values will be above zero and others will be less than zero, balancing each other out and giving a sum of zero. Instead, we square (multiply by themselves) the values in column three to obtain the values in the final column. These values are always positive. Finally we add them all together, divide the number of texts minus 1 (giving 9) then find the square root. The square root of a number is the number which multiplied by itself gives the original number. For example, 10 is the square root of 100 because 10 x 10 = 100. The same final value of 0.06243619 can be found if we put the list of proportions of long words for the texts in a list called `long`, then type the command `sd(long)`.

2.3 The Normal Distribution

The following diagram was based on code provided by statology.org/plot-normal-distribution-r. Imagine we have a large number of texts with a mean readability score of 100 with a standard deviation of 10. If they are normally distributed, we see the characteristic bell-shaped curve shown in Figure 2.1. Here we see that the largest number of texts have a readability score of the mean value, 100. We also see that the curve is symmetrical, with half the documents having readability scores above the mean, and half the documents having readability scores below the mean. A characteristic of the normal distribution is that about a third of the scores will fall between one standard deviation below the mean and one standard deviation above the mean, in our case with readability scores between 90 and 110. About 95 per cent of the texts have scores within two standard deviations of the mean (here between 80 and 120), and only about one in a thousand will have readability scores outside three standard deviations from the mean (less than 70 or more than 130). A text may be assigned a z score according to how many standard deviations its readability score is from the mean. A readability score may be translated to a z-score using the formula z = (readability score for that text – mean readability score) / standard deviation. Thus a text with a readability score of 115 would have z-score of (115 – 100) / 10 = 15/10 = 1.5. A text with a readability score of 92 would have a z-score of (92 – 100) / 10 = −8 / 10 = −0.8.

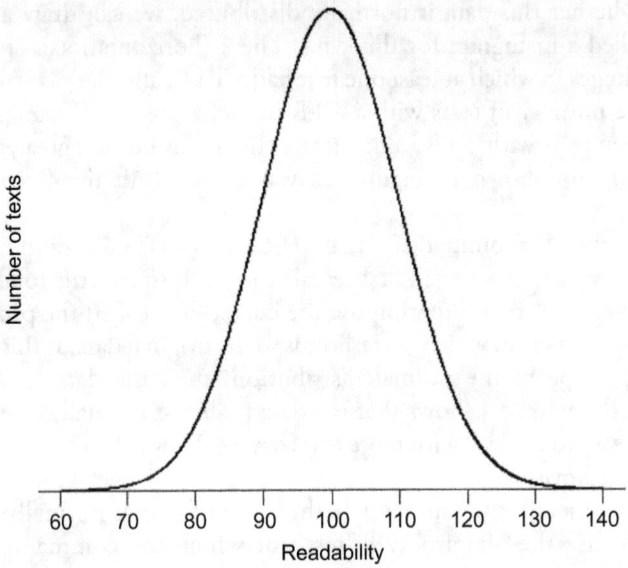

Figure 2.1 Curve assuming readability is normally distributed.

2.4 Data for the Experiment for the Type Token Ratio

Remember that the type token ratio (TTR) of a text is the number of unique words, (types) in it divided by the total number of words (tokens). We want to answer the question of whether texts with high readability tend to have lower TTR values than those with low readability. The answer to this question will be given in the form of a p-value, which is the likelihood that if high and low readability texts really had the same TTR, we would still see the difference between them in our relatively small experiment. If the TTR values were normally distributed within both the high readability and low readability groups, we could use a test from a family of 'parametric' tests called the t-test.

In the following experiment, we took a sample of thirty-nine texts where the number of words was at least 100. The TTR for each text in turn was as follows:

```
0.571 0.696 0.752 0.528 0.718 0.716  0.693 0.706 0.728
0.673 0.569 0.662 0.680 0.700 0.716  0.664 0.671 0.667
0.650 0.750 0.683 0.604 0.743 0.721  0.634 0.704 0.673
0.745 0.638 0.770 0.605 0.607 0.717  0.657 0.675 0.733
0.579 0.607 0.745
```

To see whether this data is normally distributed, we can draw a type of graph called a histogram for this data. The x (horizontal) axis shows the various ranges in which at least one text had a TTR, and the y (vertical) axis shows the number of texts with a TTR in each range. For example, there are thirteen texts with TTR values greater than 0.65 but not greater than 7. The histogram shown in Figure 2.2 was drawn with the R command `hist(ttr)`.

Using the R commands `hist(ttr, prob=T)` and `lines (density(ttr))` we can first rescale the y axis so that the total shaded area is equal to 1, then superimpose the curved line called the probability distribution function which corresponds to the original data. If this curve is the same shape as the normal distribution, then the data is normally distributed. Figure 2.3 shows that the data is almost normally distributed, but is skewed to the left, with more texts having TTR values below the peak value than above.

A more objective measure of whether a set of data is normally distributed is to use the Shapiro-Wilk test, for which the command in R is `shapiro.test(ttr)`. This returns a p-value of 0.126, which is more

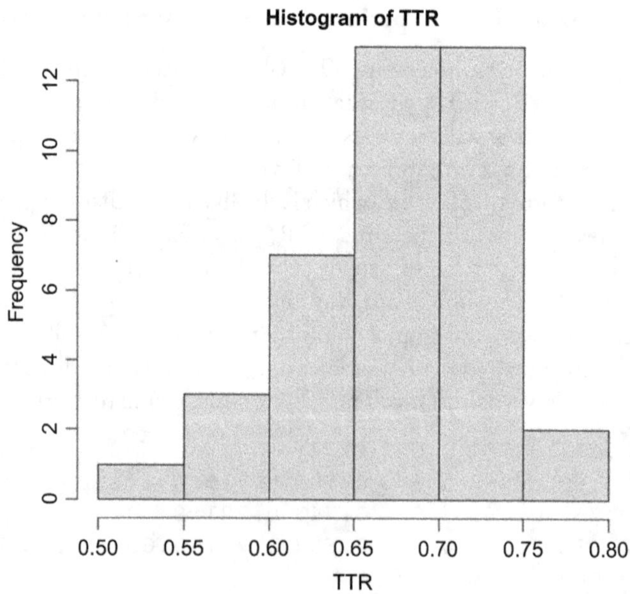

Figure 2.2 Histogram showing the non-normal distribution of TTR.

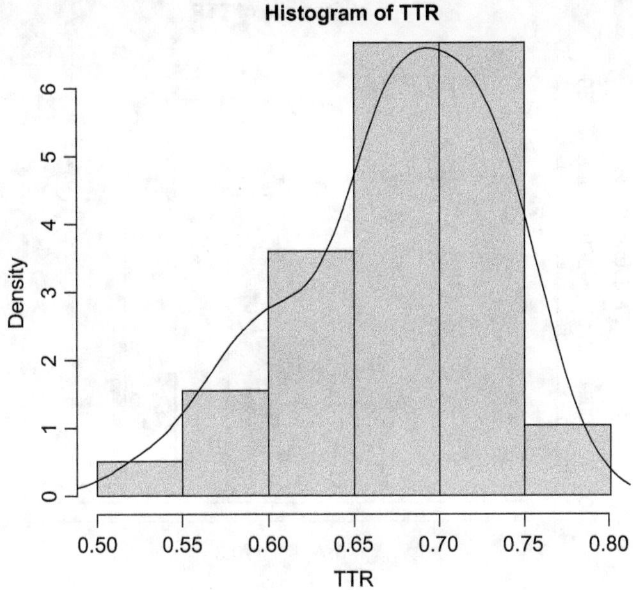

Figure 2.3 Probability distribution function for TTR.

than the arbitrary but widely used cut-off point of 0.05, suggesting that there is no significant difference between the probability distribution function we obtained and a normal distribution. This means that according to this small experiment, we could assume that the data was normally distributed, and use a so-called parametric test such as the t-test for independent samples to see whether one group of texts (such as those with high or low readability) differ from another in terms of TTR. However, TTR in general is not normally distributed. If we look at the histogram for the TTR values for a large set of data consisting of 2583 texts, we see it is strongly skewed to the left, as shown in Figure 2.4.

The Shapiro-Wilk test returns a p-value of less than 2.2×10^{-16}, a very small value which is much less than 0.05, meaning that TTR in general is definitely not normally distributed. Thus to answer our question of whether TTR is more in high or low readability texts, we should use a non-parametric test called the Mann-Whitney test. We should also use non-parametric tests if we are using small data sets, such as the thirty-nine texts used in the experiment described in Section 2.5.

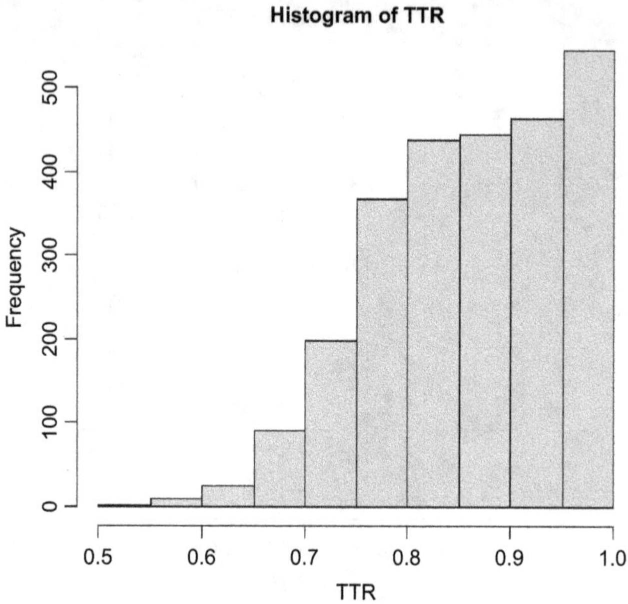

Figure 2.4 Histogram of TTR for the entire set of texts.

2.5 The Mann-Whitney Test

Imagine we ran a small experiment comparing the TTR of just five documents, two of which have high readability and the other three have low readability. When we rank the documents by TTR, there are ten possibilities: the highly readable documents have ranks (1 and 2), or (1 and 3), (1 and 4), (1 and 5), (2 and 3), (2 and 4), (2 and 5), (3 and 4), (3 and 5) or (4 and 5). The sums of the ranks for these possibilities are 3, 4, 5, 6, 5, 6, 7, 7, 8 and 9 respectively, giving a mean of 6 and a standard deviation of 1.825. The mean μ can be calculated exactly by the formula $n_S (n_S + n_L + 1) / 2$, where n_S and n_L are the number of texts in the smaller and larger groups respectively – 2 and 3 for this example. This formula applies for groups of all sizes. Similarly, there is an approximate formula for the standard deviation σ of the rank sums, which is more accurate for larger groups:

$$\sigma = \sqrt{n_L \mu \div 6}$$

Using these two formulas for the larger sample of Table 2.2, where the number of texts with high readability is 12 and the number of texts with low

Table 2.2 *Stepwise calculation of the Mann-Whitney test*

Low Readability (n=27)		High Readability (n=12)
Rank	TTR	Rank
1	0.528	
2	0.569	
	0.571	3
4	0.579	
	0.604	5
6	0.605	
7.5	0.607	
	0.607	7.5
9	0.634	
10	0.638	
11	0.650	
	0.657	12
13	0.662	
	0.664	14
15	0.667	
	0.671	16
17.5	0.673	
	0.673	17.5
19	0.675	
	0.680	20
21	0.683	
22	0.693	
23	0.696	
24	0.700	
	0.704	25
	0.706	26
27.5	0.716	
27.5	0.716	
29	0.717	
30	0.718	
31	0.721	
	0.728	32
33	0.733	
	0.743	34
35.5	0.745	
35.5	0.745	
37	0.750	
38	0.752	
39	0.770	
Sum = 780		Sum = 212

readability is 27, we get a mean rank sum of 12 (12 + 27 + 1) / 2 = 240. This is compared with the actual rank sum we obtained of 212, which we will call T. The standard deviation σ of all possible rank sums with these group sizes is $\sqrt{27 \times 240 \div 6} = 32.863$.

We now calculate a z-score using the formula z = (T – μ) / σ = (212 – 240) / 32.863 = –0.852. To find the probability of obtaining a z-score of this magnitude or greater, we consult a table of the normal distribution such as the one in Altman (1991: 518). Here the p value corresponding to a z-score of 0.85 (the closest value in the table) is 0.3953. This method works well when there are more than about ten texts in each of the high and low readability groups, since T is normally distributed for larger samples. For smaller samples, tables such as Table B10 in Altman (1991) can be used.

We can compare this result that we have worked out by hand with a very similar result obtained by running the experiment on the R programming language. We can input the TTR ratios of all the documents with low readability as follows:

```
low = c(0.528, 0.569, 0.579, 0.605, 0.607, 0.634, 0.638,
0.650, 0.662, 0.667, 0.673, 0.675, 0.683, 0.693, 0.696,
0.700, 0.716, 0.716, (0.717, 0.718, 0.721, 0.733, 0.745,
0.745, 0.750, 0.752, 0.770)
```

and the documents with high readability as follows:

```
high = c(0.571, 0.604, 0.607, 0.657, 0.664, 0.671, 0.673,
0.680, 0.704, 0.706, 0.728, 0.743)
```

and then run the Mann-Whitney test as shown below:

```
wilcox.test(low, high, paired = F)
```

The `'paired=F'` denotes that the individual texts in the high and low readability groups have no special one-to-one relationship with each other. No text in the low readability group is specifically related to any member of the high readability group. If they were paired in such a way, we would need another test called the Wilcoxon test, which would be called by

```
wilcox.test(low, high, paired = T)
```

The output gives a p value of 0.3953, which is very close to the value we calculated by hand. Both these values are greater than 0.05, so in this small experiment there is no significant difference in the TTR between texts of high and low readability. This would suggest that TTR is not a good criterion for inclusion in a readability measure.

2.6 Spearman Test

Spearman's rank correlation ρ (rho) is the non-parametric counterpart of the Pearson product-moment correlation coefficient. We will use it to compare the ranks (rather than the actual values) of the data for disease incidence and information complexity, for documents pertaining to each of the twelve disease types in Chapter 7. We want to see whether there is a significant correlation between these two variables. For diseases with higher incidence, do we tend to see documents with higher information complexity?

Spearman's rank correlation coefficient ρ is given by the formula

$$\rho = 1 - \frac{6\sum d^2}{n^3 - n}$$

n is the number of different disease types that we are considering, which is twelve. Thus $n^3 - n$ is (12 × 12 × 12) – 12 which is 1716. $\sum d^2$ is derived from Table 2.3. In the first column we list all twelve disease types, then in column 2 we put their respective incidence rankings. Since documents about influenza have the greatest incidence, we put a 1 for influenza in the incidence ranking column. Documents about influenza have only the highest complexity, so we put the value 11 in the information complexity column in the row for influenza. The difference between column 2 and

Table 2.3 *Linguistic complexity of Chinese health information on the country's leading infectious diseases*

Disease	Incidence ranking	Information complexity ranking	d	d^2
Influenza	1	11	−10	100
Hand, foot, and mouth disease	2	10	−8	64
Diarrhoea	3	3	0	0
Syphilis	4	2	2	4
Hepatitis	5	8	−3	9
Mumps	6	1	5	25
Gonorrhoea	7	5	2	4
Dysentery	8	9	−1	1
HIV / AIDS	9	7	2	4
Brucellosis	10	12	−2	4
Dengue fever	11	6	5	25
Haemorrhagic fever	12	4	8	64
				$\sum d^2 = 304$

column 3 for influenza is now 1 minus 11, which is -10. This value is written in the d (difference) column, and the value squared (-10 x -10 = 100) is written in the d^2 column for influenza. The same calculations are done for each of the other eleven disease types. Finally, we add together all twelve values in the d^2 column, to obtain the value of $\sum d^2$ which 304. 6 $\sum d^2$ is thus 6 x 304 which gives 1824. Substituting the values for 6 $\sum d^2$ and $n^3 - n$ into the formula for Spearman's ρ, we obtain

$$\rho = 1 - \frac{1824}{1716} = -0.063$$

Tables exist for converting the value of ρ into a p-value, such as table A10 in Butler (1985). Reading the row for n = 12 (as we are considering documents describing each of twelve disease types) and the column for a significance level of 0.05 for a two-tailed test, we see the value 0.587. Since the absolute (ignoring the sign) value of ρ is 0.063 is less than this, the correlation between incidence ranking and information complexity ranking is not statistically significant at the p = 0.05 level.

Spearman's ρ can also be calculated using the R programming language. The ranked data are collated into lists as follows:

```
incidence =c(1,2,3,4,5,6,7,8,9,10,11,12)
complexity = c(11,10,3,2,8,1,5,9,7,12,6,4)
```

It is also possible to put the raw data into the incidence and complexity lists, as the final answer will be the same. The Spearman test is then run as follows:

```
cor.test(incidence, complexity, method='spearman')
```

With the following output:

Spearman's rank correlation rho

```
data: incidence and complexity
S = 304, p-value = 0.8517
alternative hypothesis: true rho is not equal to 0
sample estimates:
        rho
-0.06293706
```

As we saw with the hand calculation, ρ (rho) is about -0.0629. We do not need to use tables this time, as we are given an exact p-value of 0.8517. This is much greater than the arbitrary cut-off point of 0.05, so the correlation between incidence and text complexity is not significant.

We cannot say that as one increases, so does the other, or that as one increases, the other decreases. They seem to be relatively independent of one another.

2.7 The Kruskal-Wallis Test

The Kruskal-Wallis test is an extension of the Mann-Whitney test. It is used in similar circumstances, except where we have three or more groups of data to compare instead of just two. As with the Mann-Whitney test, we record the raw data and then the ranks of the data, with the highest value ranked 1, the next highest value ranked 2, and so on. In this small example, we have taken the first ten documents in a dataset which contains original Chinese information on environmental and health promotion from the China Disease Control Centre (CDC) and translated Chinese on similar topics from the World Health Organization (WHO) and the Merck Manual of Diagnosis (MSD) Consumer Edition (https://www.msdmanuals.com/en-au/home) websites.

The documents were characterised by a measure of linguistic complexity, the average number of strokes per character. In this example we have exactly ten documents per author, but in general the groups need not be all of equal size. However, they should be independent, where for example the first CDC document has no particular relation with the first MSD text and the first WHO text. If the texts are related across authors, where for example the first texts are all on one topic, the second texts all on another topic and so on, then the Friedman test should be used.

The data may be tabulated as follows:

The sum of the ranks for the WHO documents is more than the sum of the ranks for the MSD data, which in turn is greater than the sum of the ranks for the CDC data. This suggests that fewest strokes are found per character in the WHO data, followed by the MSD data, and finally the CDC data has most strokes per character. The purpose of the Kruskal-Wallis test is to determine whether these differences are statistically significant. The Kruskal-Wallis formula is as follows (Field, 2000: 237):

$$H = \frac{12}{N(N+1)} \sum_{i=1}^{k} \frac{R_i^2}{n_i} - 3(N+1)$$

N is the total number of texts in the experiment, across all three authors, which is 30, so

$$\frac{12}{N(N+1)} = \frac{12}{30 \times 31} = \frac{12}{930}$$

The summation symbol Σ denotes that we must add together all our values for R_i^2/n_i, starting from the first (when i = 1) to the third (when i = k = 3), which is the number of author groups. The three R_i values are those in the bottom row of Table 2.4, and the three n_i values are the numbers of texts in each author group (ten in each case). Thus

$$\sum_{i=1}^{k} \frac{R_i^2}{n_i} = \frac{137 \times 137}{10} + \frac{156 \times 156}{10} + \frac{170 \times 170}{10} = 7255.7$$

N is the total number of texts across all author groups, so 3(N + 1) = 3 (30 + 1) = 93. Now we can calculate an overall value of H, which is:

$$H = \frac{12}{930} \times 7255.7 \times 93 = 0.6219$$

To determine statistical significance, H may be looked up in a table of the Chi-squared distribution, such as Table A7 in Butler (1985). Looking across the row for two degrees of freedom (the number of author groups minus one) and down from the column for a significance level of 0.05, we find a value of 3.84. This is rather higher than our H value of 0.6219, so the differences between the three author groups was not statistically significant.

Table 2.4 *Linguistic complexity of Chinese health information (average number of strokes per character) from three sources: China CDC, MSD, WHO*

CDC Raw data	CDC rank	MSD raw data	MSD rank	WHO raw data	WHO rank
7.111	28	7.423	18	7.386	21
7.677	9	7.94	3	7.556	14
6.705	30	7.315	25	7.878	4
7.128	27	7.321	24	7.521	15
7.975	2	7.394	19	7.5	16
7.654	12	7.574	12	7.003	29
7.797	5	7.495	17	7.39	20
7.649	11	8.116	1	7.372	22
7.717	8	7.671	10	7.785	6
7.757	7	7.311	26	7.363	23
	Sum = R_1= 139		Sum = R_2 =156		Sum = R_3 = 170

Using the same data, the Kruskal-Wallis H value can be calculated using the R statistical programming language. The data is read from a table in the following format, where the two columns have the headers 'author' and 'strokes.' All three authors are represented in the first column, and the individual texts are in the second column.

```
author   strokes
cdc   7.111
cdc   7.677
cdc   6.705
cdc   7.128
cdc   7.975
cdc   7.654
cdc   7.797
cdc   7.649
cdc   7.717
cdc   7.757
msd   7.423
msd   7.94
msd   7.315
msd   7.321
msd   7.394
msd   7.574
msd   7.495
msd   8.116
msd   7.671
msd   7.311
who   7.386
who   7.556
who   7.878
who   7.521
who   7.5
who   7.003
who   7.39
who   7.372
who   7.785
who   7.363
```

To read the data into a file in R called str10, we can use the following syntax:

```
str10 = read.table(file=file.choose(), header = T)
```

The Kruskal-Wallis test is run as follows:

```
kruskal.test(strokes~author, data=str10)
```

which gives the following output:

```
      Kruskal-Wallis rank sum test
data: strokes by author
Kruskal-Wallis chi-squared = 0.62194, df = 2, p-value =
0.7327
```

Once again, we get an H value (called Kruskal-Wallis chi-squared here) of 0.62194. This time we do not need any lookup tables to determine statistical significance, as the programme gives a p-value of 0.7327 automatically. This is much more than 0.05, so the differences in the number of strokes per character used by the three sub-corpora of China CDC, MSD and the WHO in this small experiment are not statistically significant.

2.8 Dunn Test

Here we describe an extended version of the small experiment described in Section 2.7. Once again we wish to determine whether the number of strokes per character used by each of the three authors (CDC, MSD and WHO) differs significantly. This time, instead of just ten texts per sub-corpus, we use 234 texts for CDC, 394 for MSD and 352 for WHO. The mean number of strokes per character was found to be 7.868 for CDC, 7.856 for MSD, and 7.711 for WHO. This data was found by reading the dataset into a file called `strokes_all`, and using the following syntax:

```
sum(strokes_all$author=='cdc')
```

to which the response was 234, and

```
mean(strokes_all$strokes[strokes_all$author=='cdc'])
```

to which the response was 7.867526. Thus, the mean number of strokes per character was least for WHO, meaning the WHO texts had the simplest writing style. However, we still needed to find whether the differences between the authors in terms of strokes per character were statistically significant. Once again, we used the Kruskal-Wallis test with the following syntax:

```
kruskal.test(strokes~author,data=strokes_all)
```

The resulting output was as follows:

```
     Kruskal-Wallis rank sum test
data: strokes by author
Kruskal-Wallis chi-squared = 41.148, df = 2, p-value =
1.161e-09
```

This time, using a much larger dataset, we get a highly significant p-value, which is much less than 0.05. The scientific notation 1.161e-09 translates to the very small value of 0.00000000161. However, this only tells us that the differences in strokes per character across all three authors is statistically significant, but we would still like to know which pairwise differences (CDC and MSD, CDC and WHO, or MSD and WHO) were responsible for the significance of the differences across all three authors. For this we used the Dunn test, which is also available in R, with the following syntax:

```
dunn.test(strokes_all$strokes, strokes_all$author)
```

The output is as follows:

```
 Kruskal-Wallis rank sum test
data: x and group
Kruskal-Wallis chi-squared = 41.1482, df = 2, p-value = 0
                              Comparison of x by group
                                   (No adjustment)

Col Mean-|
Row Mean |    cdc   msd
---------+-----------------of
     msd | 1.099458
         |   0.1358
         |
     who | 5.663711 5.276357
         |  0.0000* 0.0000*

alpha = 0.05
Reject Ho if p <= alpha/2
```

If we look at the table at the centre of the output, we see two values in the row for MSD and the column for CDC. The top value of 1.099458 is a statistic specific to the Dunn test called Dunn's z. This translates to the p-value immediately below of 0.1358, which is more than the suggested cut-off point suggested in the last two lines of 0.05 / 2 = 0.025, showing that the difference in the number of strokes per character between MSD and CDC is not statistically significant. However, if we look at the p-values for the pairwise comparisons between CDC and WHO, and MSD and WHO, we see that they are approximately 0, which is much less than our cut-off point of 0.025. Thus, the differences between these two pairs of sub-corpora is highly statistically significant.

2.9 Regression

We have looked at the Mann-Whitney test, which can tell us if a linguistic feature (such as TTR) is more prevalent in one group of texts (such as high readability texts) than another (such as low readability texts). Another way of finding out how one textual characteristic varies with another is regression. Regression tells us how much one variable increases or decreases when the other is increased by a certain amount. With the Pearson product-moment regression test, the two variables to be compared are not described by whole numbers corresponding to categories, but so-called real numbers which are actual values of the data which can be described by decimal numbers. Thus we will not describe readability as 'high' or 'low', but as exact values on the scale. Using an imaginary set of thirty-five texts, we will examine the relationship between the number of unique monosyllabic words in a text and its readability.

Figure 2.5 is a scatterplot, where each small circle corresponds to a single text (so there are thirty-five small circles in all). For each text, we can read off the

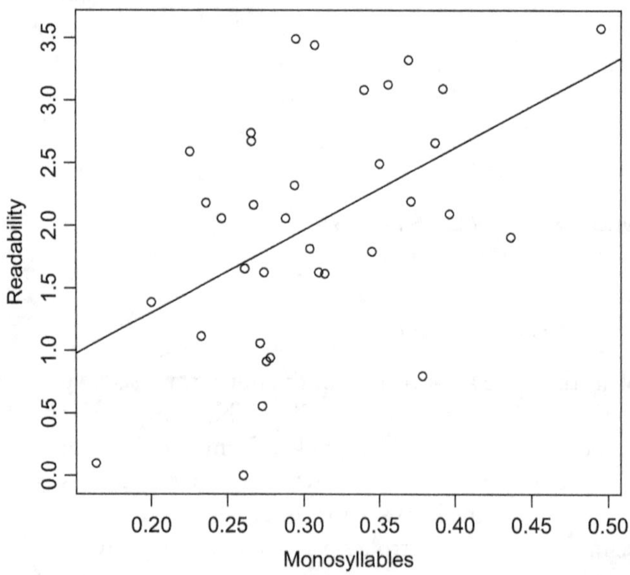

Figure 2.5 Readability as a function of the proportion of monosyllables.

proportion of unique monosyllables on the horizontal axis and the readability on the vertical axis. The straight line on the scatterplot is the line of best fit, the straight line which is closest to all the circles. In fact, it is the sum of the squares of the differences between the readability score on the straight line and the actual readability of the texts which is minimised. The straight line is called the regression line, and in this case it has a formula: readability = (6.60681 × proportion of unique monosyllabic words) – 0.02129. The -0.02129 part is called the intercept: the estimated readability of a text with no unique monosyllables. The 6.60681 value is the slope of the line: in general, the readability score is about 6.6 times the proportion of unique monosyllables in the text.

The following R commands were used to produce the scatterplot:

```
plot(monosyllables, readability)
```

was used to produce the basic graph, then to produce the regression line we used

```
res = lm(readability ~ monosyllables)
```

followed by `res` to calculate the coefficients (slope and intercept). The output is in the following format:

```
Call:
lm(formula = readability ~ monosyllables)
Coefficients:
  (Intercept) monosyllables
    -0.02129            6.60681
```

Finally we used `abline(res)` to draw the regression line on our graph.

If two variables vary exactly with each other, such as in the hypothetical case where the readability score was exactly six times as much as the value of a linguistic feature, we say we have a correlation of 1. In such a case, all the small circles would be situated exactly on the regression line. If we had such a perfect correlation where the regression line sloped downwards (so the more the value of the linguistic feature, the lower the readability score) we say we have a correlation of -1. If there was absolutely no relation between the linguistic variable and the readability score, the correlation coefficient would be 0. In cases where we have a general trend upwards, where the regression line slopes upwards but the circles do not fit exactly on the regression line, the correlation coefficient will be more than 0 but less than 1. Conversely, if the regression line slopes downwards, but the circles are scattered on either side of the line, we have a correlation coefficient of between 0 and -1. Using the R command:

```
cor.test(monosyllables, readability)
```

we find that the correlation coefficient in this example is about 0.481, and there is a corresponding p-value of about 0.0035, which is less than 0.05 so the relation between the proportion of unique monosyllables and the readability score in these thirty-five texts is statistically significant. We can also do these calculations by hand, as described in the following paragraphs. First, we fill in the values in Table 2.3, where the first column consists of the proportions of monosyllables in each of the thirty-five texts in turn. We call this set of values x. The corresponding readability scores are in column 2. We call these values y. Columns 3 and 4 are the values in the first and second columns respectively squared, i.e. multiplied by themselves. In the final column we have the values in the first column multiplied by those in the second column. The bottom row shows the sums of the values in each column, Σx, Σy, Σx^2, Σy^2 and Σxy. The sums can be combined in the following formula (Butler, 1985:144), where N is the number of texts:

$$r = \frac{N\sum xy - \sum x \sum y}{\sqrt{\{N\sum x^2 \sum (\sum x)^2\}\{N\sum y^2 \sum (\sum y)^2\}}}$$

Substituting the sums in the formula with the actual values of the sums in Table 2.3 we obtain:

$$r = \frac{(35 \times 22.53307) - (10.72 \times 70.08)}{\sqrt{\{(35 \times 3.44512) - 10.72^2\}\ \{(35 \times 170.8368) - 70.08^2\big)\}}}$$

$$r = \frac{788.6574 - 751.2576}{\sqrt{(120.5792 - 114.9184)(5958.288 - 4911.206)}}$$

$$r = \frac{37.3998}{76.9891} = 0.4857$$

which is very similar to the value of 0.4809 obtained using `cor.test` on R. The correlation coefficient r can be translated to a significance value using look-up tables such as table A9 in Butler (1985:180). For a two-tailed test using over thirty text samples, the corresponding p-value is less than 0.01, and thus there is a statistically significant relation between the proportion of unique monosyllables and the readability score.

Table 2.5 *Stepwise calculation of Pearson's product-moment regression coefficient*

Proportion of monosyllables (x)	JTRMS Readability score	x^2	y^2	Xy
0.295	3.49	0.087025	12.1801	1.02955
0.294	2.31	0.086436	5.3361	0.67914
0.345	1.79	0.119025	3.2041	0.61755
0.304	1.81	0.092416	3.2761	0.55024
0.350	2.49	0.122500	6.2001	0.87150
0.371	2.19	0.137641	4.7961	0.81249
0.436	1.90	0.190096	3.6100	0.82840
0.265	2.67	0.070225	7.1289	0.70755
0.369	3.32	0.136161	11.0224	1.22508
0.271	1.06	0.073441	1.1236	0.28726
0.260	0.00	0.067600	0.0000	0.00000
0.288	2.05	0.082944	4.2025	0.59040
0.314	1.61	0.098596	2.5921	0.50554
0.307	3.43	0.094249	11.7649	1.05301
0.387	2.66	0.149769	7.0756	1.02942
0.164	0.09	0.026896	0.0081	0.01476
0.278	0.94	0.077284	0.8836	0.26132
0.310	1.62	0.096100	2.6244	0.50220
0.340	3.08	0.115600	9.4864	1.04720
0.495	3.57	0.245025	12.7449	1.76715
0.396	2.08	0.156816	4.3264	0.82368
0.378	0.79	0.142884	0.6241	0.29862
0.392	3.09	0.153664	9.5481	1.21128
0.356	3.12	0.126736	9.7344	1.11072
0.236	2.18	0.055696	4.7524	0.51448
0.246	2.05	0.060516	4.2025	0.50430
0.261	1.65	0.068121	2.7225	0.43065
0.265	2.73	0.070225	7.4529	0.72345
0.274	1.62	0.075076	2.6244	0.44388
0.225	2.58	0.050625	6.6564	0.58050
0.233	1.11	0.054289	1.2321	0.25863
0.267	2.16	0.071289	4.6656	0.57672
0.273	0,55	0.074529	0.3025	0.15015
0.200	1.39	0.040000	1.9044	0.27600
0.275	0.91	0.075625	0.8281	0.25025
$\Sigma x = 10.72$	$\Sigma y = 70.08$	$\Sigma x^2 = 3.44512$	$\Sigma y^2=170.8368$	$\Sigma xy = 22.53307$

Table 2.5 can also be used to find the slope of the regression line, using a method described by Altman (1991:311). Let S_{xx} be $\Sigma x^2 - (\Sigma x)^2/N$ and S_{xy} be $\Sigma xy - \Sigma x \Sigma y/N$. Then the slope of = regression line, b = S_{xy} / S_{xx}. In our case, $S_{xx} = 3.44512 - (10.72)^2/35 = 0.161737$, and $S_{xy} = 22.53307 - (10.72 \times 70.08 / 35) = 1.068567$. Thus b = 1.068567 / 0.161737 = 6.606818 which accords very well with the value we obtained using R. The intercept a is found using the relation $a = \bar{y} - b\bar{x}$, where $\bar{y} = \sum y/N = 2.002286$, which is the mean readability score of our thirty-five texts. $\bar{x} = \sum x/$ N = 10.72 / 35 = 0.3062857. Thus a = 2.002286 – (6.606818 x 0.3062857) = -0.02128788, which again is very similar to the value we obtained with R.

Thus we have derived a simple readability formula:

Readability score =(6.606818 x proportion of unique monosyllables) – 0.02128788.

2.10 Multiple Regression

In the previous section we described the development of a simple readability measure using simple linear regression. With this measure, the readability score depended on a single variable, the proportion of unique monosyllables in the text. Most real readability measures depend on more than one variable, such as average word length in characters and number of difficult words. Here we are going to develop a readability measure which incorporates up to four predictor variables, namely the number of words, the TTR, the number of syllables per word and the number of proper nouns. The technique is called multiple linear regression, and can be performed on R in a similar way to simple linear regression. Assuming that the data for each text (we are going to use all 2,582 texts used for the work on Japanese translation described in Chapter 5) have been read into tables with an initial header with the name of the data, we can use the following syntax:

```
res = lm(formula = readability ~ numberofwords +
typetokenratio + syllablesperword +
numberofpropernouns)
```

followed by

```
summary(res)
```

then the key part of the output is as follows:

```
Coefficients:
                    Estimate Std. Error t value Pr(>|t|)
(Intercept)         4.042225 0.377514 10.707 < 2e-16 ***
numberofwords      -0.011721 0.001634 -7.174 9.49e-13 ***
typetokenratio      1.525186 0.367503 4.150 3.43e-05 ***
syllablesperword   -1.381125 0.086761 -15.919 < 2e-16 ***
numberofpropernouns -0.227496 5.181206 -0.044 0.965
---
Signif. codes: 0 '***' 0.001 '**' 0.01 '*' 0.05 '.' 0.1 ' ' 1
```

We see that the intercept is about 4.042, so a hypothetical text with no words, a TTR of 0, no syllables per word and no pronouns would have a readability score of this value. However, for real texts, the intercept value of 4.042 is reduced by about 0.0117 per word in the text. It is increased by about 1.525 times the TTR, reduced by about 1.381 times the number of syllables per word, and also decreased by about 0.227 times the number of pronouns in the text. However, we must also look at the final column of the output, the one headed Pr(>|t|) which contains p-values for each predictor variable. The predictor variables with p-values of less than 0.05 are marked with one or more asterisks, so since the number of pronouns has a p-value more than 0.05 (and is not marked with any asterisks), this variable can be dropped from the model. Thus our final readability score estimate is:

$$\text{Readability score estimate} = 4.042 - (0.177 \times \text{number of words}) + (1.525 \times \text{type-token ratio}) - (1.381 \times \text{syllables per word}).$$

Another part of the R output tells us something about the accuracy of our prediction model (or readability formula). A residual value for an individual text is the difference between the actual and predicted value of the readability score for that text. In a few cases our model is very inaccurate, as in the two worst cases our prediction was either –6.0974 too high or 5.7003 too low. However, we can also look at the first and third quartiles (labelled 1Q and 3Q respectively). The first quartile is the residual value which is lower for one-quarter of the texts, and higher for the other three-quarters. The third quartile is the residual value which is higher for one-quarter of the texts, and lower for the other three-quarters. The inter-quartile range (IQR) is the difference between the first and third quartiles, and thus provides a measure of spread which encompasses half the texts. Our results show that half the texts have residuals less than about 0.7 (plus or minus) and thus our readability score predications were within about 0.7 of the actual values.

```
Residuals:
    Min       1Q   Median       3Q      Max
-6.0974 -0.7107 -0.0314  0.7013  5.7003
```

2.11 Step Method Using Akaike's Information Criterion

A related method of deciding which predictor variables to add to our readability measure uses the Akaike Information Criterion (AIC) which is an estimate of prediction error produced by a statistical model to help us decide which ones to keep (Johnson, 2008:91–93). The method is to start with the assumption that all the texts have the same intercept value for their readability scores, and this does not depend on any of the predictor variables. We do this by including (readability ~ 1) in the R syntax for the whole procedure. We also make the initial assumption here that our formula can include at most the four predictor variables we looked at in the previous section, namely number of words, TTR, syllables per word and number of pronouns. Of course we could start with another maximal set of predictor variables if we wanted. We start the R programme for the step procedure with the command:

```
res = step(lm(readability ~ 1),readability ~
numberofwords + typetokenratio + syllablesperword +
numberofpropernouns)
```

The output is shown below. The first two lines show that we start by assuming that all the texts have the same readability value as the intercept, and this has an AIC of 1,384.09. Later we will add or delete predictor variables, if doing so can reduce the AIC. The next six lines show the effect of adding one of the predictor variables to the model. The one which will be most effective in reducing the AIC is syllables per word, which will reduce it to 1,028.1. The first 'step:' statement shows we have added syllable per word to the model, so the readability score estimation now depends on syllables per word as well as the intercept. We then see another block of output which shows the effect of adding or removing predictor variables, either adding a new variable or removing the one we already have. The plus signs show the effect of adding a variable, while the minus signs show the effect of removing one. At this second step, the most effective option in terms of reducing the AIC is to add the variable number of words. Now the AIC is 796.89, and our model now estimates readability as a function of both syllables per word and number of words.

At the third step we can make a small reduction to AIC to 781.69 by adding type-token ratio. At the final step, the best thing we can do is do nothing. The <none> entry shows that the AIC will remain the same if we neither add or remove any variable, while the values below show that any action, either adding number of proper nouns or removing any of the variables added in previous steps, will increase the AIC again. Thus we should do nothing, and keep our final model where the readability estimation depends on syllables per word, number of words, and TTR (as well as the intercept), which is the solution we found for the p-value method in the previous section.

```
Start: AIC=1384.09
readability ~ 1
                       Df  Sum of Sq     RSS        AIC
+ syllablesperword      1     570.86  3839.0     1028.1
+ numberofwords         1     570.73  3839.1     1028.2
+ typetokenratio        1     414.55  3995.3     1131.2
+ numberofpropernouns   1       9.49  4400.4     1380.5
<none>                                4409.9     1384.1

Step: AIC=1028.14
readability ~ syllablesperword
                       Df   Sum of Sq     RSS        AIC
+ numberofwords         1      331.60  3507.4     796.89
+ typetokenratio        1      284.82  3554.2     831.11
<none>                                 3839.0    1028.14
+ numberofpropernouns   1        2.80  3836.2    1028.26
- syllablesperword      1      570.86  4409.9    1384.09

Step:  AIC=796.89
readability ~ syllablesperword + numberofwords
                       Df  Sum of Sq          RSS       AIC
+ typetokenratio        1      23.29       3484.1    781.69
<none>                                     3507.4    796.89
+ numberofpropernouns   1       0.00       3507.4    798.89
- numberofwords         1     331.60       3839.0   1028.14
- syllablesperword      1     331.73       3839.1   1028.23

Step: AIC=781.69
readability ~ syllablesperword + numberofwords +
typetokenratio
```

	Df	Sum of Sq	RSS	AIC
<none>			3484.1	781.69
+ numberofpropernouns	1	0.00	3484.1	783.69
- typetokenratio	1	23.29	3507.4	796.89
- numberofwords	1	70.07	3554.2	831.11
- syllablesperword	1	342.98	3827.1	1022.12

2.12 Logistic Regression

In regression, we often speak of the predictor variables as independent variables, and the outcome variable as the dependent variable. We have looked at multiple regression with continuous dependent variables. Continuous here means that the variable can take any value, including those with digits after the decimal point. In contrast, categorical variables are whole numbers used to describe categories of data. In the simplest case, we might just have two categories, 0 and 1, to denote the presence or absence of some condition (Altman, 1991:351) such as 0 to denote texts with high readability and 1 to denote texts with low readability. When the outcome variable is categorical, we cannot use multiple linear regression, but we can use the related method of logistic regression. Rather than predicting for example a readability score as in linear regression, we predict the logit function of p, which is how probable it is that a text falls into the 1 category. The expression p / 1 – p is called the odds ratio, which might be the probability of a text being of low readability divided by the probability of it being of high readability. The logit function is the natural logarithm (logarithm to the base e, a function available on most scientific calculators) of the odds ratio:

$$logit(p) = log_e\left(\frac{p}{1-p}\right)$$

With linear regression, the continuous variable for predicted readability score was calculated as the sum of the intercept b_0 plus each of the values for the predicting features x_i multiplied by slopes of their regression lines b_i. In logistic regression, this sum becomes the value of the logit function, as follows:

$$log_e\left(\frac{p}{1-p}\right) = b_0 + b_1x_1 + b_2x_2 + \ldots + b_kx_k$$

If we call this quantity x, we can find the probability p with the expression:

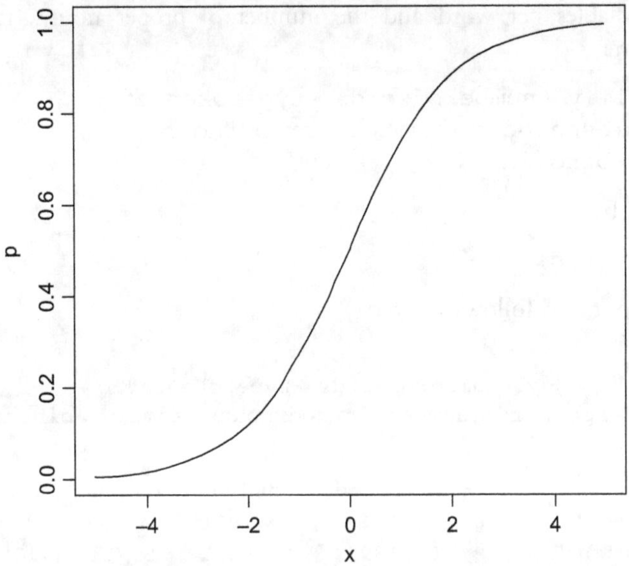

Figure 2.6 Sigmoid function relating logit to probability of low readability.

$$p = \left(\frac{e^x}{1 + e^x}\right)$$

e is a mathematical constant like π. While x can take any value, p will always be in the range 0 to 1 (Verzani, 2005:345–346). If $p > 0.5$ the text is more likely to be of low readability, while if it is less than 0.5 it is more likely to be of high readability. A graph which converts x values into p values is shown below in Figure 2.6. The 'S'-like shape of the graph is called a sigmoid. It was produced using the `invlogit()` function in the 'LaplacesDemon' package in R. See https://search.r-project.org/CRAN/refmans/LaplacesDemon/html/logit.html

Logistic regression is one of a class of models called generalised linear models, which are fit in R using the glm() function. The syntax is similar to that for linear regression, but we also must specify that "family = gaussian" for logistic regression. In the following experiment, the original readability scores are transformed to categorical data by giving all texts with a readability score above 2.5 a category of 1, and all others a category of 0. Assuming that the text being high or low readability depends at most on number of words,

TTR, syllables per word and the number of proper nouns, the commands are:

```
res = glm(y ~ numberofwords + typetokenratio +
syllablesperword + numberofpropernouns,
family=binomial)
```

followed by

```
summary(res)
```

The output is as follows:

```
Call:
glm(formula = y ~ numberofwords + typetokenratio +
syllablesperword + numberofpropernouns, family = binomial)

Coefficients:
                     Estimate  Std. Error  z value  Pr(>|z|)
(Intercept)          -3.21967   0.71981    -4.473  7.71e-06 ***
numberofwords         0.01890   0.00331     5.711  1.12e-08 ***
typetokenratio       -1.85223   0.70221    -2.638  0.00835 **
syllablesperword      2.35142   0.17511    13.428   <2e-16 ***
numberofpropernouns   2.01736  10.34087     0.195   0.84533
-
Signif. codes: 0 '***' 0.001 '**' 0.01 '*' 0.05 '.' 0.1 ' ' 1
```

The output is very similar to multiple linear regression, with the asterisks in the final column indicating that the intercept, number of words, TTR and syllables per word are all statistically significant, and should be retained in the model. On the other hand, the number of proper nouns, with a z-score of 0.84533, which is more than the arbitrary cut-off point of 0.05, can be dropped from the model. Thus our final readability measure is

$$log_e\left(\frac{p(lowreadability)}{1-p(lowreadability)}\right) = -3.21967 + (0.01890 \times numberofwords)$$
$$-(1.8523 \times typetokenratio) + (2.35142 \times syllablesperword)$$

2.13 Link with Machine Learning

Once we have built the logistic regression model for our readability data, we can use it to predict the readability (high or low, with or without and associated probability) of new texts, as yet unseen at the time of building the model. If we call the set of texts used to create the model the training data, we can use it to make predictions about the so-called testing data, which is the new set of documents that we want to classify.

Vidhi Chugh (https://www.datacamp.com/tutorial/logistic-regression-R) describes five steps we should take if we use logistic regression as a method of machine learning. First we must split all our data into testing and training sets, with typically 80 per cent of the tests in our training set and 20 per cent in our testing set. Second we should train (or fit) the model, which is what we have done in Section 2.9, where we have both reduced a maximal set of predictor variables into the set of predictors which significantly predict the category of a text, and also found the extent to which each of the predictors influences the categorisation. The third step is to make predictions for the texts in the training set. We saw how to do this in Section 2.9, where we can use our readability formula and the sigmoid function in Figure 2.6 to predict the probability of each text being either of high or low readability. The fourth step is to evaluate the model's performance, and the final step is to fine-tune the model by what is called hyperparameter estimation. In the evaluation of classifier performance, a process called cross-validation is often used. The training set is randomly split into k equally sized portions called 'folds', and if for example we use ten portions we refer to ten-fold cross validation. Here we run our classification experiment ten times, each time keeping nine of them as training data, and keep the other portion as test data. For each run we hold out a different portion as test data. We check that we get similar results for each run. The evaluation of the overall machine learning procedure in terms of accuracy in classifying the test set can be done by measuring the Area Under the Curve (AUC), as described in Chapter 4.

2.14 Support Vector Machines

Another example of supervised machine learning is the Support Vector Machine (SVM). Once again we show the system examples of documents with their linguistic features and their correct assignment as high or low readability. With these, the SVM learns to distinguish between them. Future texts, with no humanly assigned readability assignments can then automatically be assigned as high or low readability. The performance of SVMs is often excellent (Baayen, 2008:160) and they are often used as baselines against which other classifiers are compared. Imagine we categorise the texts by two features, such as TTR and syllables per word. We could draw a scatterplot where the points represented individual humanly classified texts, their position on the x axis being determined by their TTR and their position on the y axis being determined by the number of syllables per word. If we colour the points representing texts of high readability blue, and colour the points representing texts of high readability red, if we are lucky, we will see that blue points are all in one area of the plot, and the red points are in another area. We can then draw a line mid-way between the two sets of points to separate them. Ideally this line will be spaced as far as possible from the nearest points on either side, new points are added to the plot, and automatically classified according to which side of the line they fall on. The line separating the points is called a hyperplane (because it could be more like a sheet between points in three or more dimensions, as we will see in a minute), the space between the line and the nearest points on either side is called the margin, and the closest texts on either side are called support vectors. If we are not so lucky, and there is no straight line which can separate the texts, we can try again by changing one of the axes. For example, we could again plot TTR on the x axis, but this time plot number of words on a new axis which we will call the z axis. Now separation might be possible, but if not we can try more dimensions (See James Le, https://www.datacamp.com/tutorial/support-vector-machines-r). The process is made less computationally intensive by the so-called kernel trick, which involves complicated matrix algebra.

2.15 Conclusion

While this has by no means been a comprehensive review of statistics and machine learning, we hope that we have covered the most important methods used by Meng Ji in her experiments described in Chapters 3 to 6. While these experiments were run using the SPSS package which is convenient to use and provides extensive output, the examples of techniques provided in this chapter use the R statistical programming package because it provides more opportunity to 'look under the bonnet' and calculate intermediate results. We also included hand-worked examples of the Standard Deviation, the Mann-Whitney test and Pearson's Product-Moment Regression to aid understanding.

CHAPTER 3

Readability of Environmental Health Resources for Parental Education

3.1 Principles of Effective Health Communications

Communicating environmental health risks is a challenging yet important research topic (Lundgren & McMakin, 2018; Taylor-Clark, Koh, & Viswanath, 2007; McCallum, Hammond, & Covello, 1991; Lindell & Perry, 2003; Covello, 1992). Technically, risks can be estimated by multiplying probability times severity of harm (Boholm, Möller, & Hansson, 2015; Weinstein, 2000; Visschers, Meertens, Passchier, & De Vries, 2009). These abstract concepts can be explained to a professional audience in quantifiable terms using statistical models. Researchers and policy makers can leverage scientific research to take countermeasures and planned actions to minimise uncertainties and risks.

For general readers, however, the highly abstract communication style of scientific research poses a significant challenge in gaining an accurate understanding of the severity and likelihood of health risks (Golding, Krimsky, & Plough, 1992). In recent years, health research has increasingly focused on effective, meaningful public communication of health risks (Buller, et al. 2000; Jensen, 2008). In order to achieve better health promotion outcomes for diverse groups of people with varying reading skills, there is a need for more inclusive, accessible health communication (Kreuter & McClure, 2004; Thompson & Harrington, 2021; Elder, Ayala, Parra-Medina, & Talavera, 2009; Basch, Mohlman, Hillyer, & Garcia, 2020). As outlined in the World Health Organization's Strategic Communications Framework for Effective Communications, health communications should adhere to six principles: accessibility, actionability, credibility, relevance, timeliness, and understandability.

Accessibility means making health information available to the population via a variety of media, including printed texts, internet, radio, community television, and person-to-person communication (Berland et al., 2001; Maloney, 2005; Shatilwe, Hlongwana, & Mashamba-Thompson, 2022).

Actionable health information supports the adoption of healthy behaviours and the implementation of health policies and guidelines (Mastroianni et al. 2019; Shoemaker, Wolf, & Brach, 2014). Credibility of health information requires that messages be accurate, clear, and consistent (Sbaffi & Rowley, 2017; Eastin, 2006; Charnock, Shepperd, Needham, & Gann, 1999). The relevance of health advice, guidance, and information refers to its applicability and suitability to specific populations (Crystal & Greenberg, 2006; Gray, Klein, Noyce, Sesselberg, & Cantrill, 2005; van Pelt et al., 2015).

Timely delivery of health information is essential for empowering at-risk individuals and communities to make timely decisions concerning their health (Doubleday et al., 2021; Prorok, Iserman, Wilczynski, & Haynes, 2012; Akhlaq, McKinstry, Muhammad, & Sheikh 2016; Jajosky & Groseclose, 2004). Understanding means making health information comprehensible to the public, including those without technical expertise like medical professionals and allowing them to read and comprehend the vital health information being provided (Beaunoyer, Arsenault, Lomanowska, & Guitton, 2017; Balakrishnan, Chandy, Hseih, Bui, & Verma, 2016).

The World Health Organization's strategic health communications framework provides high-level guidance for developing and evaluating public-oriented health information. Implementing these principles requires developing and validating analytical instruments to assess the communicative effectiveness of written health information. These principles are not separate, isolated items. Rather, they are intrinsically linked. Understandability is a prerequisite to achieving other principles of effective health communication, such as the relevance, credibility, and actionability of health information.

A variety of quantitative linguistic tools have been developed to assess the readability of health information. For example, since the 1940s, quantitative readability instruments have been developed to predict the level of education that is required of a reader to comprehend a given piece of writing. With the use of readability tools, one can quickly evaluate the level of linguistic complexity of written materials. However, it remains unclear whether readability tools can be used to measure the communicative effectiveness of health information as proposed by the World Health Organization (WHO). Communicative effectiveness in this and the next chapters aligns with the WHO principles of health communication which include the understandability, credibility, relevance and actionability of health resources. Communicative effectiveness as studied in this chapter encompasses higher-level interaction between the sub-dimensions contributing to the design and delivery of health information.

Existing studies tend to measure communicative effectiveness by using readability tools as a quick solution to the assessment of public-oriented health information (Loughran & McDonald, 2014; Hagemeier-Klose & Wagner, 2009; Mcinnes & Haglund, 2011). However, there is an increasing number of studies which criticise the validity of the structural design of readability tools to evaluate the quality of written information, especially its suitability for different readerships (Friedman & Hoffman-Goetz, 2006; Bailin & Grafstein, 2001; Zamanian & Heydari, 2012; Keselman, Logan, Smith, Leroy, & Zeng-Treitler, 2008). Further research is needed to identify linguistic and textual features that are associated with the effective communication of environmental health information for distinct audiences.

This chapter examines the applicability and limitations of quantitative readability tools in predicting the likely readership of online environmental health educational resources. This assumes that environmental health educational resources from national health authorities or well-established health promotion organisations have been developed purposefully for and are well received by target audiences. These purposely developed, public-oriented educational materials exhibit linguistic, textual features that are large contributors to the effective communication of health messages. The chapter will develop binary classifiers to predict the likely readership of environmental health resources given their textual, linguistic features, or the readability of environmental health information for specific audiences.

3.2 Health Information Readability: A Quantitative Evaluation

The Flesch Reading Ease Formula was invented in 1948 by Dr. Rudolph Flesch (Flesch, 1950). An English text is assessed using this formula based on a regression model incorporating two linguistic features, sentence length in words and word length in syllables. The Flesch Reading Ease Index ranges from 0 to 100, with higher scores signalling greater ease with reading. A score below 50 is considered suitable for people with a high school education or higher. A score of less than 30 is considered complex, suitable for college graduates. The Flesch Reading Ease Formula was developed based on the hypothesis that shorter word length, measured by the mean syllable count per word, indicated easier, more familiar terms for the intended average readers. Flesch Reading Ease Index was developed in relation to Zipf's Law, which has been highly influential in psycholinguistics since the 1930s (Piantadosi, 2014). For communication convenience, Zipf's Law shows that shorter words were used more frequently than longer words. Hence, short words were regarded as easier to comprehend (Kanwal, Smith, Culbertson, & Kirby, 2017).

Formula 3.1 Flesch Reading Ease Formula

$$\mathbf{RE = 206.835 - (1.015 \times ASL) - (84.6 \times ASW)}$$

ASL: Average Sentence Length (the number of words divided by the number of sentences)
ASW: Average number of syllables per word (the number of syllables divided by the number of words)

Recent studies using large-scale language corpora have challenged Zipf's Law. A study by Piantadosi, Tily, & Gibson (2011) shows that word length can better be predicted by the amount of information conveyed by a word, rather than its frequency in a large corpus. They found that there was a linear relationship between the length of a word and the information conveyed by that word, which they approximated by using the mean negative log probability of the tokens of that word in a large corpus. However, researchers did not find a correlation between word length and its frequency in the corpus. The researchers tested this finding in ten languages and concluded that shorter words are not necessarily more frequent than long words as predicted by Zipf's Law. Word length was determined by the average information content of a word rather than its frequency.

Zipf's hypothesis that shorter words are more frequent, more familiar, and thus easier to comprehend for average readers led to the development of the Flesch Reading Ease Index (Flesch, 1950, 1952). In two scenarios, this poses problems for health text assessment. First, unfamiliar words, like medical abbreviations and jargon, can be more difficult to understand than frequently used, long words in everyday speech; second, for non-native speakers of English, such as international tertiary students, it is often easier for them to understand formal, more complex English words than colloquial, shorter words frequently used by native speakers (Ji, Liu, & Hao, 2021). Flesch Reading Ease Index is widely used as a convenient tool for health professionals to assess the difficulty levels of original English written materials, despite its limitations for evaluating the suitability of the material for different readers, especially readers with limited English proficiency (Table 3.1).

There have been numerous studies using the Flesch Reading Ease Index for assessing the readability of written materials for the public. The researchers found, however, that the mean scores of written materials

Table 3.1 *Flesch Reading Ease Index interpretation*

Reading Ease reading scores	Difficulty	Education level
0–30	Very difficult	Postgraduate
30–50	Difficult	Undergraduate
50–60	Fairly difficult	Year 10–12
60–70	Standard	Year 8–9
70–80	Fairly easy	Year 7
80–90	Easy	Year 6
90–100	Very easy	Year 5

developed for the public were often much lower than the desired level, for example, Year 8 or below, signifying significant reading barriers for people with an average education level of Year 8 or below (Varela-Centelles et al., 2015). From an internet sample of paediatric patient education materials for parents and caregivers of young children, D'Alessandro, Kingsley, and Johnson-West found that the average Flesch Reading Ease score of these materials was 57.0 (95 per cent confidence interval: 52.1, 65.1), which requires a minimum of Year 10 education. Considering the average educational level in developing countries is lower than that of developed countries, this consistently higher readability difficulty poses a significant barrier to the public's access to critical environmental health information. Nivera et al. (2017) examined pamphlets on how to survive natural disasters for vulnerable Filipinos. The Flesch Reading Ease scores were 58.4 for topics on wind- and water-related disasters, such as typhoons, flash floods, storm surges, and tsunamis; and 64.6 for self-protection amidst earthquakes. As a result, the intended readers in the Philippines must have a level of education equivalent to Year 10 in English-speaking countries to understand environmental education materials in English.

During the following decades, the Gunning Fog Index developed by Robert Gunning, an American publisher, became another popular readability tool (Gunning, 1969). As with Flesch Reading Ease scores, it was based on the hypothesis that the two key linguistic features that helped predict text difficulty were the frequency of complex words and the number of words comprising three or more syllables. Unlike the Flesch Reading Ease Index, which provides continuous scores between 0 and 100, the Gunning Fog Index provides graded reading ease levels; higher grades indicate greater levels of difficulty. In general, Grade 12 is considered suitable for people with Year 12 or higher education; For people with education at or below the college level, grade 16 or higher is considered extremely complex. The lowest Gunning Fog Index score is 0.4, which occurs only when a text contains words that are less than three syllables long. The Gunning Fog Index has no upper limit. In contrast, the upper limit of the Flesch Reading Ease is 121.22, which is based on a list of monosyllabic words, and there is no lower limit.

Formula 3.2 Gunning Fog Index Formula

$$\textbf{Grade Level} = \textbf{0.4}\ (\textbf{ASL} + \textbf{PCW} \times \textbf{100})$$

ASL: Average Sentence Length (the number of words divided by the number of sentences)
PCW: Percentage of complex words of three or more syllables (the number of complex words divided by the number of words)

Peter et al. analysed twenty-six online sources of information related to prenatal microarrays and exome sequencing. They found that the mean Gunning Fog Index score was 15.4 (standard deviation, 2.0), suggesting that these online health resources for parent prenatal education require minimal university education to be understandable. Wong and Levi compared five readability tools to examine the understandability of paediatric otolaryngology-related patient education materials in leading online sources such as the top ten US News and World Report-ranked children's hospitals, the top five Doximity-ranked paediatric otolaryngology fellowships, and the American Academy of Otolaryngology-Head and Neck Surgery. The mean Gunning Fog Index scores of these resources were 13.1 (95 per cent confidence interval: 12.31, 13.83, min: 10.2, max: 15.5). The results were consistent with previous studies that evaluated the understandability of health educational materials for parents and found a high level of education, sometimes tertiary, as a threshold to understand the materials (Table 3.2).

SMOG Grading–A New Readability Formula was published in 1969 by G. Harry McLaughlin (McLaughlin, 1969). A clinical psychologist from London, McLaughlin used the initialism 'SMOG' not only to refer to his birthplace London, but also to pay homage to Robert Gunning who created the Gunning Fog Index. More importantly, the naming highlighted the importance of the concept of polysyllabic words for the SMOG Index. McLaughlin's SMOG index simplified earlier versions of readability tools by measuring reading difficulty solely based on polysyllabic words. McLaughlin made this purposeful, innovative decision to

Table 3.2 *Gunning Fog Index interpretation*

Gunning Fog Index	Difficulty	Education level
16	Very difficult	College graduate
15, 14, 13	Difficult	Undergraduate
11 to 12	Fairly difficult	Year 11–12
10	Fairly difficult	Year 10
9	Standard	Year 9
8	Standard	Year 8
7	Easy	Year 7
6	Easy	Year 6

replace earlier readability designs with a formula that is easier to calculate, faster, and more accurate. Earlier readability formulas based on regression analysis added unnecessary complexity to the estimation of readability levels, he argued. The SMOG Grade Index reduced the two previously used linguistic factors as sources of reading difficulty, word length and sentence length, to one, that is, polysyllabic words.

McLaughlin observed that word length and sentence length interact as sources of semantic and syntactic difficulty. When word length was altered in two sentences of varying lengths, the reading difficulty changed differently between harder, longer sentences and easier, shorter sentences. Based on the number of polysyllabic words alone, he discovered a law that can accurately predict the length of passages in syllables. At the time, this was a highly innovative approach to assessing the readability of written content. It challenged the traditional linguistic formulation of reading difficulty, which combines semantic and syntactic complexity as if they were completely unrelated attributes. Using the polysyllabic word analytical unit, introduced by Robert Gunning, McLaughlin introduced a more intuitive method of assessing reading proficiency compared to previous formulas. McLaughlin developed a set of simple, step-by-step guides to approximating readability grades. SMOG grade is roughly equal to the minimum level of education needed to comprehend the text. As its inventor envisioned half a century ago, the SMOG Index today is the most simple, convenient way to measure readability, which can be used with fingers or brain power alone.

A study by Mandic, Rudd, Hehir, & Acevedo-Garcia (2010) investigated literacy barriers to understanding materials on the legal rights of students with disabilities and their parents. To determine the readability of procedural safeguards documents distributed by U.S. state departments of education, they used the SMOG Index. For parents of children with disabilities, they adapted the SMOG tool to fit the principle of clear legal writing and applied the revised formula to assess the readability of these legal materials. Of all materials examined from fifty-one states, only about 6 per cent (from three states) had mean SMOG scores between 10 and 12, meaning that parents must have a minimum high school education in order to understand the materials. On the other hand, more than half (55 per cent) (from twenty-eight states) of the materials had mean SMOG scores between 13 and 16, which were equivalent to university education. In the remaining 39 per cent of materials from twenty states, the mean SMOG score was 17 or higher, which is equivalent to university graduates or professionals.

Although readability formulas are simple and convenient, there are also some limitations associated with these tools. Health authorities, for example, have expressed concerns about the validity and suitability of these tools for evaluating health information quality from the perspective of readers. The Health and Human Services' Agency for the U.S. Healthcare Research and Quality raised concerns about the correct use and interpretation of readability tools. Readability tools, for example, assume that word length and sentence length are the only factors that affect reading difficulty. It has been overlooked that the understandability of health information is dependent upon many factors, including lexical familiarity, clarity, and structural cohesiveness. In addition, readability tools can only produce grade-level scores. Readability tools cannot answer questions such as whether health information is effective or understandable for different audiences. Consequently, readability tools are more suited to grading texts rather than assessing the communicative effectiveness of health information or the prediction of the suitability of health information for specific audiences.

According to the latest definition of effective communications by the WHO, a people-centred or target-audience-oriented approach to health information quality assessment is more appropriate and effective. The purpose of this study is therefore to develop automatic classifiers to predict whether a certain online environmental health educational text is more suitable for the general public or a more specific reader group such as parents of young children. For this purpose, a large corpus of materials developed for general public communication and parental environmental health education was developed and used as the basis for the corpus analysis. Environmental health texts intended for the general public were used as reference materials to contrast them with those designed for parents of young children and help them to develop essential environmental health literacy.

In the development of automatic binary classifiers to predict the intended audience of environmental health information, readability measures were used as predictor features. The performance of the binary classifiers was measured in terms of the overall prediction accuracy or the area under the curve (AUC), the accuracy of prediction of environmental health texts as suitable for parents or the sensitivity of classifiers, and the accuracy of prediction of environmental health texts as intended for general public or the specificity of classifiers. The results show that when using readability tools to evaluate environmental health information suitability, the higher the sensitivity, the higher the false positivity, and the higher the specificity, the higher the false negativity. This finding suggests that health information communicative effectiveness for specific audiences as defined by the WHO requires the development of new analytical measures and tools to supersede existing readability tools, which will be discussed in detail in the next chapter. The subsequent sections of this chapter will discuss the various steps taken to develop binary regression models to predict the suitability of environmental health resources for parents, in comparison with the written materials developed for a general audience.

3.3 Construction of the Corpus of Environmental Health Materials

Among popular quantitative methods for evaluating educational materials is logistic regression. Readability tools typically use multinomial logistic regression (MLR) to predict outcomes of rank or ordinal values like school grades. There was a practical reason for developing binary logistic regression (BLR), rather than MLR models in this study. For developing models, it is necessary to collect large quantities of high-quality health materials specifically developed for a certain reader group (in the hundreds at least) in order to accurately predict how likely an environmental health text is to be suitable for that reader group. With small datasets, automatic models are prone to bias and are less generalisable. In this study, the search on the internet for environmental health materials was restricted to those developed for the public, instead of health or medical professionals. This practice was to ensure that the environmental health information to be gathered was from credible, reliable sources and was also of reduced difficulties.

Through extensive internet searches, two large sets of environmental health texts were gathered which were for the general public and parents of young children. The quantity of materials intended for other readers or at-risk populations was insufficient for developing quantitative models. When developing regression models for these two reader groups, i.e., the general public and parents, BLR was deemed a more suitable option because environmental health texts for these groups were in sufficient quantities.

There were over 2.2 million words in the corpus containing online environmental health information, including 1,091,528 words in the sub-corpus containing educational resources designed for a general audience, and 1,076,569 words in the sub-corpus containing parent-oriented information. In the general public corpus, the top twenty sources of information were WebMD (124,892 words), Healthline Media (116,651 words), Centers for Disease Control and Prevention (104,812 words), Mayo Clinic (95,102 words), National Institute of Environmental Health Sciences (91,037 words), U.S. Environmental Protection Agency (66,972 words), American Society of Clinical Oncology (60,366 words), Department of Health Victoria (Australia) (51,756 words), Radiological Society of North America (49,141 words), National Institutes of Health, National Library of Medicine (45,101 words), Cleveland Clinic (42,289 words), Canadian Cancer Society (23,164 words), American Lung Association (19,852 words), MedicineNet (18,330 words), U.S. Air Quality Index (16,127 words), Society of Nuclear Medicine and Molecular Imaging (14,211 words), Cancer Council Victoria (Australia) (12,037 words), Health Physics Society (11,539 words), International Atomic Energy Agency (10,785 words), and Macmillan Cancer Support (10,124 words).

A further forty sources of information were included in the public-oriented subcorpus. The size of environmental health texts collected from these sources was under 10,000 words: New Zealand Dermatological Society (9,983 words), Cancer Council Australia (8,984 words), Centers for Disease Control and Prevention, Emergency Response (7,225 words), World Health Organization (4,610 words), American Academy of Family Physicians (4,241 words), Department of Health, UK (3,183 words), National Heart, Lung, and Blood Institute (1,940 words), Asthma and Allergy Foundation of America (1,370 words), The Environmental Factor, National Institute of Environmental Health Sciences (1,066 words), American College of Medical Toxicology (973 words), and so on. In selecting information from these reputable websites, the intended audience was the key selection criterion. Public-oriented environmental health information was retained. Materials intended for professionals, specialists, or for research purposes were not included because their purpose was not to engage the public or communicate about environmental health issues. There were fewer sources for parent-oriented environmental health texts. For parents and caregivers of children and teenagers, the following sources offered credible environmental health information: Nemours Children's Health (911,953 words), National Institute of Environmental Health Sciences (101,123 words), American Academy of Paediatrics (46,065 words), Centers for Disease Control and Prevention (7,312 words), The Society for Paediatric Dermatology (3,328 words), Nationwide Children's Hospital (2,945 words), US Environmental Protection Agency (2,220 words), and The Society for Paediatric Dermatology (1,623 words).

A topic analysis based on latent Dirichlet allocation (LDA) was carried out in Python on the two sets of environmental texts developed for public communications and parental environmental education to understand the variety of contents in these materials (Jelodar et al., 2018). The result is presented in Table 3.3. The model identifies, extracts, and summarises a predefined set of topics that provide important clues of the underlying contents of large quantities of unclassified documents (Jacobi, van Atteveldt, W., & Welbers, 2015). The purpose of deploying topic modelling is to ascertain whether important thematic variation exists between the two sets of corpus texts, i.e., public- versus parent-oriented environmental health texts. If the result of topic modelling reveals important contrasts between the two sets of corpus texts, it is likely that the preference for certain thematic topics will impact on the performance of the binary classifiers. By contrast, if the two sets of environmental health information resemble each other in the distribution of texts across the ten topics, it is likely to be other linguistic and textual features, rather than the contents, which matter more for the effective communications of environmental health risks for distinct audiences. Table 3.3 shows that topic modelling extracted ten thematic topics. These are abstract, underlying themes of the whole corpus of environmental health materials. Despite the different sources of information, there are important overlaps between public- and parent-oriented environmental health materials. Materials in both sets are mostly related to Topics 0 and 8, suggesting that thematic variability is unlikely to affect the outcome of automatic classification.

As shown in Table 3.4, the content of texts clustering around each topic can be interpreted by examining the keyword lists. By analysing the keyword list, we can infer that texts in Topic 0 are most related to water safety and toxic chemicals such as lead as well as child protection. This

Table 3.3 *Topic modelling of the data collected*

Topics	0	1	2	3	4	5	6	7	8	9	Total
Parents	**454**	3	3	5	0	0	3	0	**938**	0	1406
	32%	0.2%	0.2%	0.3%	0	0	0.2%	0	**66.7%**	0	100%
Public	**398**	27	10	23	0	4	40	70	**373**	30	975
	41%	2.8%	1%	2.3%	0	0.4%	4%	7%	**38%**	3%	100%

Table 3.4 *Key words for each topic*

Topic 0	health, water, lead, people, child, home, information, work, time, problem, school, find, clean, include, source
Topic 1	risk, cancer, study, skin, age, year, participant, high, exposure, report, increase, include, factor, case, analysis
Topic 2	soil, fertilizer, treatment, plant, increase, high, application, result, content, concentration, study, effect, organic, growth, yield
Topic 3	heat, temperature, hot, stress, day, increase, condition, high, time, wave, cold, effect, exercise, rate, study
Topic 4	gene, sample, expression, show, figure, analysis, control, cell, level, datum, perform, compare, group, protein
Topic 5	cell, tumour, melanoma, expression, cancer, skin, protein, increase, induce, show, gene, mutation, role, response, growth
Topic 6	air, pollution, study, exposure, effect, level, health, pm, high, increase, model, mortality, pollutant, risk, disease
Topic 7	cancer, lung, patient, treatment, study, clinical, stage, include, tumour, high, disease, survival, screening, rate, year
Topic 8	doctor, child, body, symptom, skin, blood, call, treatment, people, test, problem, kid, type, infection, baby
Topic 9	radiation, dose, exposure, effect, mouse, injury, day, group, animal, induce, irradiation, treatment, damage, increase, study

topic is covered extensively by both the public-oriented and parent-oriented environmental health resources: general texts (398 articles – 41 per cent) and parent-oriented (454 articles – 32 per cent). The keywords of Topic 8 suggest that texts classified to Topic 8 are related to diseases associated with skin conditions – during the data collection process, texts referring to skin cancer were related to excessive exposure to radiation and sunlight. Both public-oriented and parental environmental health resources had extensive coverage of this topic: general public (373 articles – 38 per cent), and parental (938 articles – 66.7 per cent). There is some limited coverage of Topic 6, 7 and 9 in public-oriented environmental materials but not in parental environmental education resources, suggesting a thematically more varied approach to environmental health promotion among the general public than among parents. The keywords included in these topics suggest they are related to human health impact of air pollution (Topic 6), lung cancer detection and treatment (Topic 7), and the health impact of radiation exposure from laboratory testing on animals (Topic 9). The result of topic modelling indicates that thematic variation is unlikely to be a significant contributor to the classification of the environmental health resources collected in terms of their intended audience, i.e., general public or parents of young children. Next, we will develop automatic classifiers to predict the likely intended readership of environmental health information.

3.4 Using Readability Tools to Predict Readerships of Environmental Resources

As discussed earlier, readability tools have been widely used as standard instruments for quantitative evaluations of health education resources for many decades. The data were analysed using the IBM SPSS Statistics (version 26) and readability tools as binary logistic classifiers. Through adjusting their thresholds, which were school grades, or continuous scores computed by readability tools, we selected some of the best sensitivity-specificity pairs for these readability-based classifiers. Among the readability tools used as binary classifiers were Flesch Reading Ease Index, Gunning Fog Index, SMOG Index and FORCAST Readability Index. Similar to the SMOG Index, the FORCAST Index is a simplified version of earlier readability formulas. While the SMOG Index measured textual complexity by counting the number of multisyllabic words, the FORCAST Index measured text reading ease by counting the number of monosyllabic words in every 150 words. In summary, the linguistic features used by readability tools to predict textual understandability include average sentence length in words and average word length in syllables (Flesch Reading Ease Index); average sentence length in words and percentage of polysyllabic words (Gunning Fog Index); averaged frequency of polysyllabic words (SMOG Index), and averaged frequency of monosyllabic words (FORCAST Readability Index).

Table 3.5 shows the results of the evaluation of the understandability of two large sets of environmental health resources. All four readability tools found a higher level of difficulty for information intended for the general public than for information intended for parents. The lowest readability score of parent-oriented materials was 11 (SD=1.6) based on the SMOG Index, which recommends that written materials be understood by parents with at least Year 11 education. Based on the Flesch Ease Reading Index, the highest score of readability for parent-oriented materials was 62 (SD=11.7), which required a minimum of Year 8 education to understand. It was nevertheless clear from the large standard deviation of the Flesch Reading Ease Index that there was considerable variation in the reading ease of parent-oriented materials. On the Flesch Reading Ease Index, the lowest readability score for general public resources was 46 (SD=15.4), and on the

Table 3.5 *Readability levels of public- versus parent-oriented environmental health materials*

Label	Intended Readers	Mean	Std. Deviation	Std. Error Mean	Education Level
Flesch Reading Ease	Parents	62	11.653	0.309	Year 8–9
	General Public	46	15.378	0.496	Undergraduate
FORCAST	Parents	10	0.800	0.021	Year 10
	General Public	11	0.880	0.028	Year 11
Gunning Fog Index	Parents	10	1.976	0.052	Year 10
	General Public	12	2.530	0.082	Year 12
SMOG Index	Parents	11	1.644	0.044	Year 11
	General Public	13	2.090	0.067	Undergraduate

SMOG Index, it was 13. Both results suggest that environmental health materials developed for general public communication require university education to be understandable.

By the FORCAST Index, Year 11 (SD=0.89) scored the highest in readability for public-oriented environmental materials The Flesch Reading Ease Index indicated that the largest gap of readability levels between the two sets of texts was between three to four years of education, and the FORCAST Index indicated that the smallest gap was only one year of high school education

Even though both sets of environmental health materials varied in terms of reading difficulty, both exceeded the Year 8 education level recommended by health authorities for public-oriented health materials to be accessible and understandable for the majority of the population. The research question worth discussing is whether a single readability formula could be utilised to predict the suitability of a certain health text for the general public as compared with narrowed reader groups, like parents and caregivers of young children. Or to put it another way, we are interested in knowing whether information suitability is an issue of readability.

3.5 Developing Classifiers to Predict the Readership of Environmental Resources

To better understand binary classification performance indicators, let us first look at some of the key terms such as area under the curve (AUC) of the receiver operating characteristic curve (ROC), sensitivity, and specificity.

Table 3.6 *Classification evaluation indicators*

Real Value	Predicted Value	
	Positive value (PV)	Negative Value (NV)
Positive value	True Positive (TP)	False Negative (FN)
Negative value	False Positive (FP)	True Negative (TN)

Sensitivity = TP / (TP + FN); **Specificity** = TN / (TN + FP)

Table 3.6 is the confusion matrix used in model classification evaluation. Sensitivity is the ratio of correctively predicted positive cases or true positive cases (TP) to all real positive cases including true positive (TP) and false negative cases (FN). Sensitivity can also be calculated by subtracting the false negative rate or the so-called type II (β) error from 1. Specificity is the ratio of correctly predicted negative cases or true negative cases to all real negative cases including true negative (TN) and false positive (FP) cases. Specificity is obtained by subtracting the false positivity or type I (α) error from 1.

Area under the curve of the receiver operating characteristic curve (AUC of ROC) is an overall model performance indicator (Zweig & Campbell, 1993). A ROC is drawn on a coordinate grid, with the horizontal axis representing Type I (α) error or false positivity calculated by subtracting specificity from 1; and the vertical axis representing sensitivity. ROC is the graphical representation of Type 1 error and sensitivity pairs under different thresholds. Better binary classifiers are indicated by smaller values on the horizontal axis and higher values on the vertical axis. An ideal model reaches the upper left corner point of (0, 1) when the model sensitivity is 1 with no false positive predictions or Type 1 error. The diagonal line represents a random prediction (AUC=0.5). Only ROCs above the diagonal line are considered valid.

Table 3.7 shows that Flesh Reading Ease Index (AUC=0.0806) has the highest ROC, followed by SMOG Index (AUC=0.791), FORCAST Index (AUC=0.779), and Gunning Fog Index (AUC=0.764). In the non-parametric (distribution free) test, all four binary classifiers based on readability tools achieved statistically significant (p<0.001) higher AUC over the 0.5 threshold. Given their overall high performance, the question is whether these classifiers can be used to reliably predict whether an environmental health text is suitable for a general audience or a parent of a young child. Classifiers with high AUC should also have high sensitivity and specificity pairs, which show how well the classifier can predict positive

Table 3.7 *Area under the curve of the receiver operating characteristic curve of binary classifiers using readability tools*

Classifiers	AUC	Std. Error [a]	Asymptotic Sig. [b]	Asymptotic 95% Confidence Interval	
				Lower Bound	Upper Bound
Flesch Reading Ease	.806	.009	.000	.787	.824
SMOG	.791	.010	.000	.772	.810
FORCAST	.779	.010	.000	.760	.798
Gunning Fog	.764	.010	.000	.745	.784

a. Under the nonparametric assumption. b. Null hypothesis: true area = 0.5

and negative outcomes, respectively. In this study, positive cases were environmental health articles written specifically for parents of young children, and negative or reference cases were environmental health materials written for the general public. For each binary classifier, we need to identify the best sensitivity and specificity pair, which can be a school grade or a continuous score, depending on the design of the readability tool.

Tables 3.8, 3.9, 3.10, and 3.11 show the sensitivity and specificity pairs of the four binary classifiers. In the left column, 'Positive if greater than or equal to', are the threshold values of each readability tool. When the readability score computed for a text is equal to or larger than a threshold score, the text will automatically be classified as a positive case, or a text related to environmental health that is appropriate and relevant for parents of young children. The readability score calculated for a text that is less than a threshold value will be classified as a negative case, that is, the text is more suitable for a general reader who does not have explicit responsibility for child rearing and parenting. It is apparent that across all classifiers, sensitivity decreases as specificity increases, and vice versa. It is desirable for a classifier to have a balance between sensitivity and specificity as well as a small Type 1 error. Lowering the threshold value further increases classifier sensitivity, as well as Type I error or false positivity. As a result, the binary classifier would predict more texts as suitable environmental health materials for parents of young children when considering more difficult reading levels as reference points; and more texts were mistakenly predicted as unsuitable for the public, resulting in inflated Type 1 errors. As the readability threshold value is increased, however, model sensitivity and Type 1 error decrease, while

Table 3.8 *Sensitivity and specificity pairs and thresholds for Flesch Reading Ease Index Classifier*

Positive if Greater Than or Equal To	Sensitivity	Specificity	Type 1 Error
39.5	0.829	0.593	0.407
40.5	0.809	0.636	0.364
41.5	0.783	0.669	0.331
42.5	0.752	0.703	0.297
43.5	0.729	0.729	0.271
44.5	0.704	0.759	0.241
45.5	0.684	0.785	0.215
46.5	0.662	0.812	0.188
47.5	0.637	0.835	0.165
48.5	0.603	0.851	0.149
49.5	0.574	0.872	0.128

Table 3.9 *Sensitivity and specificity pairs and thresholds for FORCAST Index Classifier*

Positive if Greater Than or Equal To	Sensitivity	Specificity	Type 1 Error
10.25	0.847	0.504	0.496
10.35	0.817	0.552	0.448
10.45	0.793	0.598	0.402
10.55	0.758	0.642	0.358
10.65	0.726	0.686	0.314
10.75	0.678	0.726	0.274
10.85	0.635	0.775	0.225
10.95	0.594	0.815	0.185
11.05	0.549	0.853	0.147
11.15	0.494	0.882	0.118
11.25	0.451	0.911	0.089

model specificity increases, along with Type II error or false negativity. Consequently, by increasing the reading ease levels as reference points, more texts will be predicted incorrectly as not suitable for parents, while more texts will be predicted correctly as suitable for public consumption.

3.6 Conclusion

In exploring the suitability of environmental health information for parental education, this chapter shows that the binary classifiers have either

Table 3.10 *Sensitivity and specificity pairs and thresholds for Gunning Fog Index Classifier*

Positive if Greater Than or Equal To	Sensitivity	Specificity	Type 1 Error
9.85	0.78	0.593	0.407
9.95	0.77	0.613	0.387
10.05	0.752	0.631	0.369
10.15	0.732	0.653	0.347
10.25	0.718	0.672	0.328
10.35	0.703	0.688	0.312
10.45	0.689	0.704	0.296
10.55	0.672	0.718	0.282
10.65	0.66	0.736	0.264
10.75	0.64	0.752	0.248
10.85	0.626	0.768	0.232
10.95	0.611	0.782	0.218
11.05	0.595	0.794	0.206
11.15	0.578	0.807	0.193

Table 3.11 *Sensitivity and specificity pairs and associated thresholds for SMOG Index Classifier*

Positive if Greater Than or Equal To	Sensitivity	Specificity	Type 1 Error
10.85	0.836	0.553	0.447
10.95	0.829	0.578	0.422
11.05	0.811	0.598	0.402
11.15	0.79	0.615	0.385
11.25	0.775	0.635	0.365
11.35	0.757	0.663	0.337
11.45	0.738	0.686	0.314
11.55	0.718	0.714	0.286
11.65	**0.7**	**0.737**	**0.263**
11.75	**0.687**	**0.757**	**0.243**
11.85	0.668	0.769	0.231
11.95	0.65	0.783	0.217
12.05	0.625	0.805	0.195
12.15	0.615	0.819	0.181
12.25	0.592	0.834	0.166

large Type 1 or Type 2 errors. These errors can have important implications in real-life contexts. Increased Type 1 errors will lead to more environmental health texts being categorised as suitable for parents that are in fact not suitable for this reader group. Consequently, if environmental health organisations used these resources, the relevance of parental environmental health education would be significantly reduced for this reader group. The lack of suitable environmental health educational resources for at-risk populations, for example, parents from disadvantaged socioeconomic backgrounds, would expose their children and themselves to more environmental health risks such as air and water pollution, toxic chemicals, nuclear radiation, extreme climatic conditions, and so on.

Allowing Type 2 errors of binary classifiers to increase will lead to more texts erroneously predicted as suitable for the public rather than parents. For environmental health education amongst parents, larger Type 2 errors will necessarily alert health authorities or health information service providers, prompting them to hire more specialised staff to conduct in-depth expert review and revision of the environmental health information that is predicted as non-suitable for parents. In situations of environmental health emergencies, this would put a strain on healthcare services, and delay the timely delivery of environmental health information for the general public. In addition, this will compromise the affordability or accessibility and timeliness of health messages, two other large principles of the WHO Strategic Communications Framework. In low-resource countries, the budget for environmental health education is often limited. In health systems that are already stretched, high rates of Type 2 errors such as those examined in this study would cause unnecessary financial burdens.

Individual circumstances and priorities in the assessment play a large role in setting thresholds for user-oriented health text assessment. This study assumes that the development of environmental health information takes place in a well-funded environment, and the priority is to achieve an optimal result of environmental health education for parents to reduce the probability that young children will be exposed to environmental health hazards or harms because of ineffective parental environmental health education. It is therefore essential to set the thresholds of binary classifiers to minimize Type 1 error while maintaining high sensitivity and specificity. Type 1 error is directly related to assessment efficiency in this study. Type 1 error rate, also known as false positivity, is the proportion of environmental health texts that would be predicted by a binary classifier as suitable for parental education but were not.

Table 3.8 shows that the best range of thresholds for the Flesch Reading Ease Index was between 42.5 and 44.5. Within this range, the sensitivity and specificity were both higher than 0.70. In this range, Type 1 error rates ranged between 0.241 and 0.291. As shown in Table 3.9, the best threshold range for FORCAST Index was between 10.55 and 10.75. Under thresholds within this range, no sensitivity and specificity pair both achieved 0.7. Their associated Type 1 errors ranged between 0.274 and 0.358. As shown in Table 3.10, the optimal reading level for people with Year 10 education is between 10.25 and 10.45 based on the Gunning Fog Index. A Type 1 error rate of 0.296 was associated with the best sensitivity-specificity pair of 0.689 and 0.704. Based on the data in Table 3.11, the best range of thresholds for SMOG Index was between 11.55 and 11.75, which corresponds to Year 11 education. From the comparison of binary classifiers based on popular readability tools, some best sensitivity-specificity pairs were Flesch Reading Ease Index at a cut-off point of 44.5: sensitivity (0.704), specificity (0.759), Type 1 error (0.241); Flesch Reading Ease Index at a cut-off point of 43.5: sensitivity (0.729), specificity (0.729), Type 1 error (0.271); SMOG Index with a cut-off point of 11.65: sensitivity (0.7), specificity (0.737), Type 1 error (0.263); SMOG Index at the cut-off point of 11.75: sensitivity (0.687), specificity (0.757), Type 1 error (0.243).

Accuracy analyses revealed some limitations of binary classifiers based on popular readability tools. After adjusting the thresholds of the classifiers measuring the reading difficulties of environmental health educational resources, we identified some best sensitivity-specificity pairs showing balanced performance of the classifiers. The limitations of classifiers with high sensitivity and low specificity include Type 1 errors or false positives. Higher Type 1 errors may confuse users of binary classifiers as automatic resource assessment tools by inflating the number of environmental health resources suitable for parental education. This would compromise the outcome and efficiency of online environmental health education for parents and caregivers of young children. For environmental health information assessment in some low-resource scenarios, classifiers with low sensitivity and high specificity may present as unfeasible, high-cost models.

The main aim of introducing quantitative or automatic assessment of information is to increase convenience and cost-effectiveness. Although these tools cannot replace expert evaluation by health professionals or educators, they provide reliable and evidence-based decision aids for facilitating the development of user-adaptive health resources. Type 2 errors, or so-called false negative rates, will be higher for classifiers with low sensitivity and high specificity. False negative rates, in our study, refer to the proportion of environmental health materials that were incorrectly classified as unsuitable for parents. This will require health organisations to engage with domain experts in order to review and revise texts classified by automatic assessment tools as unsuitable for parental environmental health education. In low-resource scenarios with limited budgets for healthcare and/or a lack of qualified health educators or domain experts, this will inevitably increase the cost of health resource development. The best models of binary classifiers examined here had sensitivity and specificity between 0.6 and 0.7, which is considered to be moderate classification performance.

Current readability tools are characterised by their simplistic linguistic models. Readability was largely determined by the length of words and sentences. There were other factors affecting cognitive and linguistic comprehension of written materials, such as textual coherence, logic clarity, and emotional engagement. Furthermore, readability tools cannot assess the suitability of health materials for various readers, as criticised by health information quality control authorities. Compared to earlier studies of automatic information assessment, natural language engineering has advanced rapidly, allowing us to develop theoretically richer, and technically more accurate evaluation models. The next chapter will use machine learning to identify new linguistic features to predict the suitability of environmental health materials for parents and caregivers of young children.

CHAPTER 4

Exploring the Suitability of Environmental Health Information for Parental Education Using Machine Learning Models

4.1 Introduction

In its Strategic Framework for Effective Health Communications, the World Health Organization (WHO) emphasises the importance of making health information understandable and relevant to different audiences. To assess the suitability of health information, many existing studies used readability formulas (Loughran & McDonald, 2014; Hagemeier-Klose & Wagner, 2009; McInnes & Haglund, 2011). However, concerns have been raised about whether different communication principles such as understandability and relevance can be reliably measured by the quantitative tools originally designed to assess readability of written materials (Friedman & Hoffman-Goetz, 2006; Bailin & Grafstein, 2001; Zamanian & Heydari, 2012; Keselman, Logan, Smith, Leroy, & Zeng-Treitler, 2008). This chapter will explore new assessment tools for the quantitative assessment of health information quality, or the suitability of environmental health information for different audiences. This chapter will develop theoretically enriched models that are more precise and cost-effective for user-centred evaluation of environmental health information quality. In this chapter, new computational models will focus on whether environmental health texts are suitable for parents rather than the general public. Logistic regression models will identify linguistic features that are important contributors to the prediction of the suitability of environmental health materials for parents and caregivers of young children, who are more likely to be affected by environmental health risks such as water pollution, excessive sun exposure, and radiation in natural and indoor environments.

The purpose of using machine learning for environmental health information evaluation is two-fold: first, machine learning models can significantly improve the accuracy of the binary classifiers discussed in the previous chapter. Evaluation of the performance of binary classifiers shows that suitability of environmental health information for parents instead of the general public cannot be accurately predicted by school grades generated by readability tools. On the one hand, increased sensitivity of classifiers comes with increased false predictivity, which can reduce the educational effectiveness of the materials. On the other hand, increasing the specificity of binary classifiers leads to increased false negativity, which implies that an increased rate of environmental health materials would be classified as unsuitable for parents when they are actually suitable for this readership. Among the practical consequences of higher false negativity are inflated costs of engaging health professionals to conduct more lengthy and costly reviews, as well as the revision of materials erroneously classified as unsuitable for parental environmental health education. In low-resource contexts whereby health professionals with skills and qualification in community environmental health communication are few, prediction by classifiers with higher false negativity can pose significant logistical challenges.

The second objective of using machine learning in this chapter is to develop linguistically enriched models to advance understanding of linguistic factors contributing to the suitability and relevance of environmental health information for different readers, in this case, parents and caregivers of young children in comparison with the general public. Existing readability tools are primarily based on two linguistic features, word length and sentence length. According to health authorities like the Agency for Healthcare Research and Quality, the simplistic approach of readability formula is not appropriate for assessing the suitability of health information for diverse users, as readability tools fail to consider the complexity of health information comprehension and individual differences. A growing body of research on health communication has suggested that a number of textual and linguistic factors can enhance the communicative effectiveness of health messages, among them semantic, sentiment, lexico-grammatical, and syntactic factors (Xie and Liu, 2022; Crossley et al., 2020; Xie, Ji, Liu, Hao, & Chow, 2021; Strekalova et al., 2017; Harvey & Koteyko, 2013; Carter, Adolphs, Brown, Crawford, & Sahota, 2007; Crawford, Brown, & Harvey, 2014; Harvey, Mahlberg, & Teubert, 2015; Kim & Fuemmeler, 2019; Matthiessen, 2013). These studies have significantly broadened the scope of earlier psycholinguistic theories that viewed health text comprehension as a lexical problem alone. Based on recent studies of health communication from a linguistic perspective, this chapter will explore linguistic features and constructs which are contributors to the automatic prediction of the suitability of environmental health information for parental education purposes.

4.2 Corpus Feature Annotation

Three popular natural language processing systems were used to annotate environmental health education texts with multidimensional sentiment, semantic, and lexico-grammatical information. Sentiment analysis was performed using the Sentiment Analysis and Social Cognition Engine (SEANCE) developed at Georgia State University (Crossley, Kyle, & McNamara, 2016; Szkody & McKinney, 2021). There are 254 core indices in the system, covering a wide range of human emotions, sentiments, social cognition, and social order. For example, words expressing dominance, longing, anger, anxiety, boredom, contempt, desperation, disappointment, disgust, dissatisfaction, pleasure, enjoyment, pride, relief, positivity, being touched, compassion, gratitude, humility, surprise, thoughtfulness, perception, comparison, evaluation, kinship, affiliation, role, power gain, power loss, authority, respect and so on. SEANCE is a popular tool in the field of natural language engineering and in the development of computational tools for information evaluation. In specialised texts, for example when discussing the impacts of environmental health harms on at-risk groups, including young children, these sentiment-related features may evoke emotional reactions in the intended audience, i.e., parents and caregivers. This study incorporates the multidimensional sentiment features provided by the SEANCE system in the development of computerised models for evaluating the suitability of environmental health materials for parents of young children versus the general public.

The semantic analysis of corpora is another important aspect of annotation. We note that some overlap exists between the UCREL Semantic Analysis System (USAS) (Rayson, Archer, Piao, & McEnery, 2004) and the SEANCE. Lexical categories covered in USAS include general or abstract terms (A), the body and the individual (B), arts and crafts (C), emotions (E), food and farming (F), government and public (G), housing (H), money (I), sports and games (K), life and living things (L), travel and transport (M), numbers and measurements (N), substances and materials (O), education (P), language and communication (Q), social actions, states and processes (S), time (T), world and environment (W), psychological actions, states and processes (X), science and technology (Y), and names or grammar (Z). There are several subcategories within each large category, and there are 453 subcategories within the twenty-one major discourse fields of USAS. A few of USAS's semantic categories are particularly relevant to the corpus analysis of environmental health educational texts such as general or abstract terms (A), the body and the individual (B), substances and materials (O), world and environment (W), social actions, states, and processes (S). To assess the suitability of health information for parental environmental health education, we therefore implemented semantic analysis in the development of computerised models.

The third corpus annotation tool used was Readability Studio (Shedlosky-Shoemaker, Sturm, Saleem, & Kelly, 2008). For measuring the complexity of written materials, it provides a comprehensive analysis of lexical, grammatical, and syntactic features: average number of sentences per paragraph, number of sentences, number of difficult sentences (containing more than twenty-two words), longest sentence, average sentence length in words, number of interrogative sentences or questions, number of exclamatory sentences, number of words, number of unique words, number of syllables per word, number of characters (punctuation excluded), number of characters and punctuation, average number of characters, average number of syllables, number of numerals, number of proper nouns, number of monosyllabic words, number of unique monosyllabic words, number of complex words containing three or more syllables, number of unique (occurring only once) complex words containing three or more syllables, number of long words containing six or more characters, number of unique (occurring only once) long words containing six or more characters, mis-spellings, repeated words, wording errors, redundant phrases, overused words, wordy expressions, cliché, passive voice, sentences beginning with conjunctions, sentences beginning with lowercase words. Numerous studies have used lexico-grammatical and syntactic features provided by Readability Studio to assess the linguistic complexity of a wide range of written materials, from education to health to media to business (Kasabwala, Agarwal, Hansberry, Baredes, & Eloy, 2012; Misra et al., 2012; Meillier, Patel, & Al-Osaimi, 2015; Shah, Yi, & Stein, 2015; du Toit, 2017; Agarwal, Hansberry, Sabourin, Tomei, & Prestigiacomo, 2013; Hansberry, Agarwal, Gonzales, & Baker, 2014). These are collectively referred to as structural features in this study. These structural features provide important information about lexical, syntactic, and phrasal complexity of written materials.

These comprehensive corpus annotation systems were developed separately, so their architectural designs have some overlap over specific annotation categories. Z99, for instance, is a classification used by the semantic tool USAS to identify words that are rarely used or not in dictionaries. As a result of the corpus analysis, it was found that the word class of Z99 in USAS exhibits significant overlap with the words that Readability Studio classified as misspellings. Furthermore, there were some overlaps between the semantic and sentiment analysis categories, particularly with respect to various types of human emotions, psychological states, and cognitive processes. As a first step in minimising the impact of possible multicollinearity on the logistic regression models to be developed, feature optimisation, reduction, and normalisation techniques were applied to identify feature sets with the least degree of interdependence or overlap.

4.3 Automatic Feature Optimisation

Figure 4.1 shows the results of automatic feature optimisation using recursive feature elimination (RFE) (Lin et al., 2012). To automate feature reduction, Zero-importance feature elimination (RZF) was used (Saarela & Jauhiainen, 2021). Before conducting RFE, the total number of linguistic features included in the corpus analysis was 390, including 247 sentiment features, 111 semantic, 32 lexical, grammatical, and syntactic features collectively called structural features. In order to develop computational models with increased generalisability, a relatively small subset of features from this extensive feature set needs to be identified. Combining overlapping features also contributes to developing linguistically more interpretable models, which is also a major objective of our study. Support vector machine (SVM) was used as the basis of recursive feature elimination for automated feature optimisation (Diederich, Kindermann, & Leopold, 2003; Zhang, Yoshida, & Tang, 2008). Cross-validation classification error (CVCE) is used as the search criterion when automatically selecting linguistic features (Kim, 2009; Braga-Neto & Dougherty, 2004). When the CVCE reaches its minimal level, the best set of linguistic features is identified. Figure 4.1 (a) to (c) illustrates the separate optimisation of sentiment, semantic, and structural linguistic features. When the CVCE reached its lowest point of 0.0861, the original sentiment feature set was reduced from 247 to 95. As well, the original semantic feature set was reduced from 111 to 104 when the CVCE reached its minimum of 0.1196. The original structural feature set was optimised from 32 to 13 with a CVCE of 0.1884 as a minimum. The last stage of the process was the joint optimisation of these three sets of linguistic features, considering that there may well exist a higher level of interaction between semantic, sentiment, and structural features. This resulted in the largest reduction of features selected from the original set of 390 to 65, representing 17 per cent of the original set. Also, the CVCE was 0.1818, the second lowest.

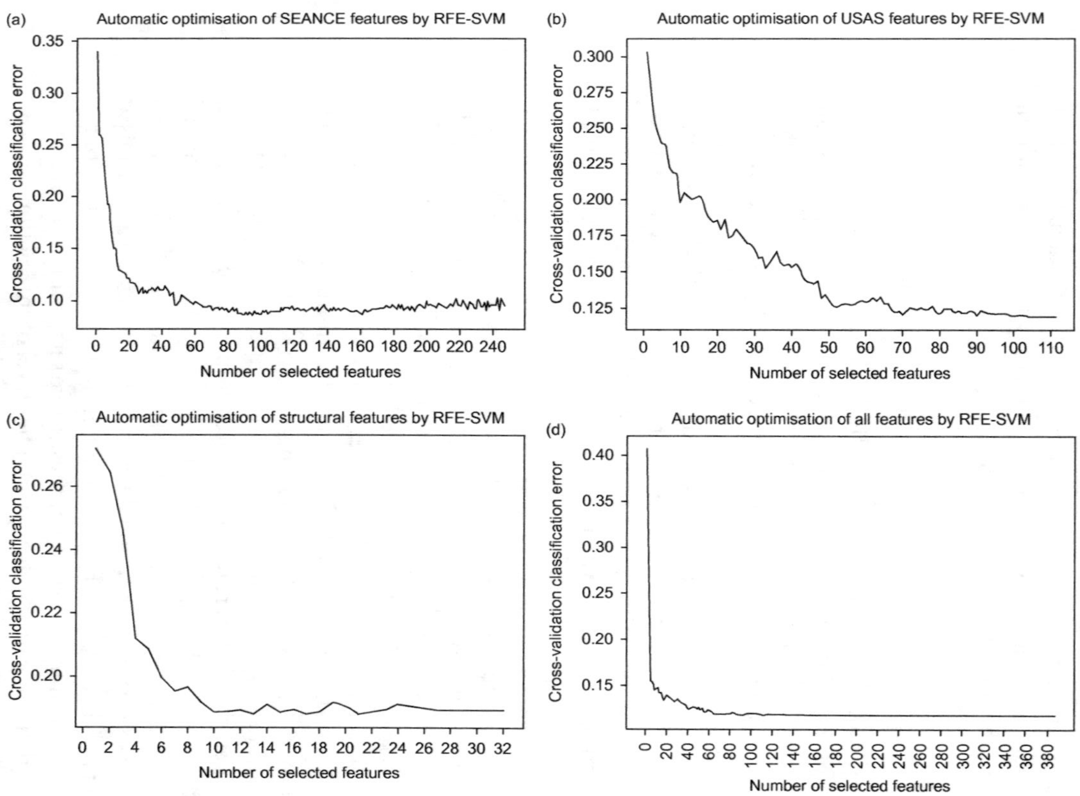

Figure 4.1 Automatic feature selection recursive feature elimination.
Cross-validation classification error (CVCE)
(a) Automatic optimisation of SEANCE features (from 247 to 95 feature, CVCE=0.0861)
(b) Automatic optimisation of USAS features (from 111 to 104 features, CVCE=0.1196)
(c) Automatic optimisation of structural features (from 32 to 13 features, CVCE= 0.1884)

4.4 Evaluation of the Performance of Machine Learning Models

The subset of public-oriented environmental health texts contained 963 articles with an average length of 1,133 words. There were 1,426 articles in the sub-corpus of parent-oriented environmental health texts, averaging 755 words per article. Texts aimed at the general public were 1.5 times longer than those aimed at parents. To facilitate the development of machine learning models, each sub-corpus was split into a training dataset of 70 per cent and a testing dataset of 30 per cent as shown in Table 4.1. As the model was a logistic regression, parent-oriented texts were labelled 1 as the outcome to be predicted, and general public-oriented texts were labelled 0, as the reference category. Logistic regression models were developed by using 70 per cent training data through fivefold cross-validation in order to reduce biases, despite the fact that logistic regression models are unlikely to have overfitting issues like other machine learning models. This is evident in the very small standard deviation associated with the mean Area under the Curve (AUC) of each model. During cross-validation, a mean AUC score was obtained, which indicated the overall performance of the model. The model's consistency and reliability were tested on the remaining 30 per cent of the dataset. In addition to assessing the accuracy of the model to predict both positive and negative cases, sensitivity and specificity were evaluated, which was discussed in-depth in the previous chapter. The goal was to identify the best models with the highest performance and the fewest features by comparing overall accuracy and outcome-specific prediction and classification accuracy.

Tables 4.2, 4.3, and 4.4 follow the same pattern of successive model comparison and selection. For each of these tables, we first evaluated the model using the original feature set as provided by the three automatic feature annotation systems; we then applied three popular feature normalisation techniques known as minmax (MM), L2 and z-score normalisation to increase classification accuracy. To reduce redundant and less effective features, two feature optimisation techniques were used successively on the

Table 4.1 *Training and testing datasets*

	Parent-oriented (1)	General public-oriented (0)	Total
Training data	992	680	1672
Testing data	434	283	717
Total	1426	963	2389

Table 4.2 *Performance of Logistic Regression (LR) classifiers with SEANCE sentiment features*

	Training data		Testing data				
LR	AUC Mean	SD.	AUC	Accuracy	Sensitivity	Specificity	Macro-F1
SEANCE 270	0.964	0.016	0.964	0.908	0.926	0.880	0.904
SEANCE 270 MM	0.967	0.015	0.970	0.925	0.938	0.905	0.921
SEANCE 270 L2	0.960	0.019	0.955	0.901	0.919	0.873	0.896
SEANCE 270 z-score	0.965	0.014	0.968	0.911	0.919	0.898	0.907
SEANCE RZF 247	0.964	0.016	0.964	0.908	0.926	0.880	0.904
SEANCE RZF 247 MM	0.967	0.015	0.968	0.923	0.940	0.898	0.920
SEANCE RZF 247 L2	0.960	0.019	0.955	0.900	0.917	0.873	0.895
SEANCE RZF 247 z-score	0.966	0.013	0.969	0.919	0.931	0.901	0.916
SÉANCE RFE 95	0.970	0.011	0.963	0.907	0.917	0.891	0.903
SÉANCE RFE 95 MM	0.970	0.011	0.965	0.902	0.915	0.883	0.898
SÉANCE RFE 95 L2	0.970	0.009	0.965	0.909	0.919	0.894	0.905
SÉANCE RFE 95 z-score	0.970	0.011	0.965	0.908	0.924	0.883	0.904

Table 4.3 *Performance of LR classifiers with USAS features*

LR	Training data		Testing data				
	AUC Mean	SD.	AUC	Accuracy	Sensitivity	Specificity	Macro-F1
USAS 115	0.931	0.009	0.930	0.880	0.915	0.827	0.874
USAS 115 MM	0.931	0.011	0.928	0.887	0.926	0.827	0.881
USAS 115 L2	0.931	0.010	0.927	0.866	0.903	0.809	0.859
USAS 115 z-score	0.931	0.010	0.929	0.890	0.940	0.813	0.883
USAS RZF 111	0.931	0.009	0.930	0.880	0.915	0.827	0.874
USAS RZF 111 MM	0.931	0.013	0.927	0.886	0.926	0.823	0.879
USAS RZF 111 L2	0.931	0.011	0.927	0.866	0.903	0.809	0.859
USAS RZF 111 z-score	0.933	0.014	0.928	0.890	0.940	0.813	0.883
USAS RFE 104	0.931	0.008	0.929	0.873	0.917	0.806	0.866
USAS RFE 104 MM	0.931	0.010	0.929	0.877	0.908	0.830	0.871
USAS RFE 104 L2	0.931	0.011	0.922	0.863	0.896	0.813	0.856
USAS RFE 104 z-score	0.931	0.011	0.931	0.876	0.906	0.830	0.869

Table 4.4 *Performance of LR classifiers with structural features*

	Training data		Testing data				
LR	AUC Mean	SD.	AUC	Accuracy	Sensitivity	Specificity	Macro-F1
Structural 33	0.896	0.010	0.902	0.840	0.880	0.777	0.831
Structural 33 MM	0.897	0.009	0.903	0.842	0.885	0.777	0.834
Structural 33 L2	0.877	0.018	0.876	0.826	0.846	0.795	0.819
Structural 33 z-score	0.897	0.009	0.903	0.844	0.887	0.777	0.835
Structural RZF 32	0.895	0.010	0.903	0.841	0.880	0.781	0.833
Structural RZF 32 MM	0.897	0.009	0.903	0.844	0.887	0.777	0.835
Structural RZF 32 L2	0.877	0.018	0.876	0.826	0.846	0.795	0.819
Structural RZF 32 z-score	0.897	0.010	0.903	0.844	0.887	0.777	0.835
Structural RFE 13	0.872	0.023	0.880	0.824	0.857	0.774	0.816
Structural RFE 13 MM	0.872	0.022	0.880	0.820	0.850	0.774	0.812
Structural RFE 13 L2	0.870	0.020	0.866	0.813	0.827	0.792	0.806
Structural RFE 13 z-score	0.873	0.022	0.880	0.822	0.855	0.770	0.813

original feature set. These techniques had little impact on the model's performance. These two procedures are known as zero-importance feature elimination (RZF) and recursive feature elimination (RFE). After applying RZF, followed by RFE, the final optimised set of features were normalised. These iterative experiments were conducted to identify the best model that has the fewest features but the most overall and outcome-specific prediction accuracy, since such models can be used to automatically assess the suitability of environmental texts for intended readers.

The process of comparing and selecting the best model annotated with multiple sentiment features is shown in Table 4.2. As many as 270 features were included in the original feature set. This model achieved a mean AUC of 0.964 on both training and testing data. According to the results, the accuracy of the prediction for positive cases, i.e., environmental health texts suitable for parental education, was 0.926, and the accuracy of the prediction for negative cases, which were environmental health materials intended for general audiences, was 0.880. AUC on training and testing data improved slightly after min-max and z-score feature normalisation, as did the sensitivity and specificity pairs. The L_2 feature normalisation resulted in a marginal reduction in model efficiency. The same pattern was observed in the next series of models (SEANCE RZF247) with a reduced feature set after automatic zero-importance feature elimination (RZF). Sentiment features were further reduced by recursive feature elimination (RFE), resulting in a series of models with the smallest sentiment features (SEANCE RFE 95). It shows the overall performance increased despite a 65 per cent reduction in features from 270 to 95. The AUC of the model (SEANCE RFE95) improved marginally from 0.964 to 0.970 on the training dataset but remained largely unchanged on the testing dataset. The sensitivity decreased from 0.926 to 0.917, while the specificity increased from 0.880 to 0.891. Using z-score feature normalisation, we were able to maintain the performance of the optimised model (SEANCE RFE 95 z-score) on the testing data to the same level as that of the original model with a large number of features (SEANCE 270): AUC (0.965), accuracy (0.908), sensitivity (0.924), specificity (0.883). By increasing the parsimony and interpretability of an optimised model, the results illustrate the significance of feature optimisation on model performance.

The comparison and selection of logistic regression models annotated with multiple semantic features are shown in Table 4.3. USAS115 is the initial model with the original full feature set (115). The mean AUC on the training data was 0.931 (SD=0.009). The AUC on the testing dataset remained unchanged. Sensitivity and specificity were 0.915 and 0.827

respectively, indicating a rather balanced model. After applying min-max and z-score feature normalisation, sensitivity increased from 0.915 to 0.926 and 0.940 respectively, while specificity either remained unchanged or dropped slightly from 0.827 to 0.813. Similar to the effects identified in Table 4.2, L_2 feature normalisation reduced the model efficiency marginally. Zero-importance feature elimination only reduced four redundant features without significant changes on the model performance. Lastly, recursive feature elimination reduced a further seven features and the optimised model (USAS RFE 104) had very similar AUC (0.873), sensitivity (0.917), specificity (0.806) on the testing data as the original model (USAS 115). Based on this finding, automatic feature optimisation led to limited improvements on the logistic regression model based on multidimensional semantic features.

In Table 4.4, logistic regression models annotated with structural features such as lexical, syntactic, and phrasal features were compared. On the training dataset, the model with the full feature set (Structural 33) had an AUC of 0.896 and on the testing dataset, it had a mean AUC of 0.902. With as few as thirty-three features, the model had a sensitivity of 0.880 and a specificity of 0.777. The min-max and z-score feature normalisations marginally improved sensitivity while maintaining specificity at the same level. After recursive feature elimination, the original thirty-three features were reduced by 60 per cent to thirteen features in the optimised feature set. The final optimised model (Structural RFE 13) had by far the smallest set of features, however, its overall performance on the testing dataset was comparable to that of the un-optimised model (Structural 33): AUC (0.824), sensitivity (0.857) and specificity (0.774). The optimised set of structural features (thirteen) contained the average number of sentences per paragraph, average sentence length, number of interrogative sentences (questions), number of characters and punctuation, number of numerals, number of monosyllabic words, number of unique monosyllabic words, number of complex (three or more syllables) words, number of unique complex (three or more syllables) words, out-of-dictionary words, overused words, wordy items, and sentences that begin with lowercase words.

Joint optimisation of all three feature sets were conducted in Table 4.5, under the hypothesis that sentiment, semantic and structural factors contributed to the suitability of written materials for parental environmental health education. The original model (All 418) contained 418 features including 270 sentiment, 115 semantic, 33 structural features. Its mean AUC on the training data was 0.957 (SD=0.007) which remained unchanged on the testing dataset. Sensitivity was 0.936 and specificity

Table 4.5 *Performance of LR classifiers with all (SEANCE + USAS + structural) features*

LR	Training data		Testing data				
	AUC Mean	SD.	AUC	Accuracy	Sensitivity	Specificity	Macro-F1
ALL 418	0.957	0.007	0.956	0.901	0.936	0.848	0.895
ALL 418 MM	0.980	0.013	0.978	0.944	0.959	0.922	0.942
ALL 418 L2	0.957	0.007	0.949	0.894	0.919	0.855	0.889
ALL 418 z-score	0.981	0.011	0.979	0.946	0.961	0.922	0.943
ALL RZF 388	0.957	0.006	0.956	0.901	0.936	0.848	0.895
ALL RZF 388 MM	0.980	0.012	0.977	0.940	0.956	0.915	0.937
ALL RZF 388 L2	0.957	0.007	0.949	0.893	0.919	0.852	0.887
ALL RZF 388 z-score	0.980	0.011	0.979	0.941	0.956	0.919	0.939
ALL RFE 65	0.956	0.011	0.954	0.900	0.919	0.869	0.895
ALL RFE 65 MM	0.961	0.008	0.951	0.894	0.936	0.830	0.888
ALL RFE 65 L2	0.957	0.010	0.943	0.882	0.910	0.838	0.875
ALL RFE 65 z-score	0.962	0.007	0.954	0.901	0.931	0.855	0.896

was 0.848, very similar to the model with the original sentiment feature sets (SEANCE 270). Min-Max and z-scores feature normalisation improved the overall model performance, as well as sensitivity and specificity. Zero importance feature elimination removed thirty redundant features without affecting the model prediction accuracy. The min-max and z-score feature normalisation techniques had comparable effects on the refined model by increasing its sensitivity and specificity to above 0.90. With a feature set of 388, it remains difficult to develop linguistically concise, interpretable models. Further feature reduction was conducted by recursive feature elimination (RFE), which reduced the original feature set by 85 per cent to sixty-five features. The final model with z-score feature normalisation (All RFE 65 z-score) achieved on the testing dataset an AUC of 0.954, sensitivity of 0.931, and specificity of 0.855. Prediction accuracy was as high as the original, non-optimised model (All 418) but with only 15 per cent of the original features.

The optimised feature set (sixty-five) contained two sentiment features: arousal, dominance; eighteen structural features: average number of sentences per paragraph, number of sentences, average sentence length, number of interrogative sentences, number of exclamatory sentences, number of words, number of unique words, number of syllables, number of characters (punctuation excluded), number of characters and punctuation, number of numerals, number of unique monosyllabic words, number of complex (three or more syllables) words, number of unique complex (three or more syllables) words, out-of-dictionary words, overused words, wordy items, sentences that begin with lowercase words; and forty-five semantic features: A1 (general, abstract terms), A10 (hiding, finding, showing), A12 (easy/difficult), A15 (safety/danger), A3 (being), A6 (comparing), A7 (probability), A9 (getting, giving), B1 (anatomy, physiology), B2 (health, disease), B3 (medicines, medical treatment), B4 (cleaning, personal care), B5 (personal belongings), F1 (food), H2 (buildings), H4 (residence), I2 (business), K5 (sports, games), L2 (living creatures), L3 (plants), M3 (land transport), M6 (location, direction), M7 (places), N1 (numbers), N3 (measurement), O1 (substances and materials generally), O3 (electrical equipment), O4 (physical attributes), S1 (social actions, states, processes), S2 (people), S3 (relationship), S4 (kin), S6 (obligation, necessity), T1 (time), T3 (age), W2 (light), W3 (geographical terms), X2 (mental actions and processes), X3 (sensory), Y1 (science, technology in general), Z3 (other proper names), Z5 (grammatical bin), Z6 (negative), Z8 (pronouns), Z99 (out of dictionary words).

Table 4.6 shows the pairwise combination of individually optimised features which included ninety-five sentimental features (SEANCE 95),

Table 4.6 *Performance of LR classifiers with multiple feature sets*

LR	Training data		Testing data				
	AUC Mean	SD.	AUC	Accuracy	Sensitivity	Specificity	Macro-F1
SEANCE95 + USAS104	0.965	0.007	0.965	0.915	0.933	0.887	0.911
SEANCE95 + USAS104 MM	0.979	0.011	0.973	0.934	0.949	0.912	0.931
SEANCE95 + USAS104 L2	0.931	0.011	0.930	0.862	0.887	0.823	0.855
SEANCE95 + USAS104 z-score	0.978	0.009	0.972	0.933	0.947	0.912	0.930
SEANCE95 + Structural13	0.884	0.017	0.942	0.876	0.883	0.866	0.871
SEANCE95 + Structural13 MM	0.976	0.011	0.976	0.933	0.940	0.922	0.930
SEANCE95 + Structural13 L2	0.870	0.019	0.867	0.813	0.827	0.792	0.806
SEANCE95 + Structural13 z-score	0.977	0.008	0.977	0.929	0.938	0.915	0.926
USAS104 + Structural13	0.952	0.011	0.953	0.891	0.915	0.855	0.886
USAS104 + Structural13 MM	0.950	0.011	0.947	0.905	0.947	0.841	0.899
USAS104 + Structural13 L2	0.957	0.009	0.949	0.895	0.919	0.859	0.890
USAS104 + Structural13 z-score	0.950	0.015	0.952	0.898	0.929	0.852	0.893
SEANCE95 + USAS104 + Structural13	0.952	0.011	0.953	0.891	0.915	0.855	0.886
SEANCE95 + USAS104 + Structural13 MM	**0.981**	**0.010**	**0.977**	**0.941**	**0.954**	**0.922**	**0.939**
SEANCE95 + USAS104 + Structural13 L2	0.957	0.009	0.949	0.895	0.919	0.859	0.890
SEANCE95 + USAS104 + Structural13 z-score	0.982	0.008	0.977	0.939	0.952	0.919	0.936

104 semantic features (USAS104) and thirteen structural features (structural 13). It shows that the best performing model was the one combining all three sets of individually optimised features with the min-max feature normalisation (SEANCE95 + USAS104 + Structural13 MM). This model achieved on the testing dataset the highest AUC of 0.977, and the highest sensitivity (0.954), and the highest specificity (0.922). However, the large number of features (212) significantly increased the complexity to use and interpret this model in both research and practical scenarios. The next section will use statistical significance as the selection criteria to further reduce the features identified and retained in the automatic feature optimisation process.

4.5 Statistical Feature Selection

A common issue with machine learning is the lack of interpretability of the features selected through the automatic process. Since this study aims to develop linguistically and statistically interpretable machine learning models, another round of further selection of linguistic features from the optimised feature set was conducted using recursive feature selection. The statistical method used was Mann Whitney test (Whitney, 1997; Li & Ge, 2009; Vold, 2006), which is a typical non-parametric test to evaluate whether the distribution of linguistic features in two sets of data is statistically significant or not at a predefined threshold (p-value). This study used effect size (η^2) of Mann Whitney U test to measure statistical significance in addition to the p-value (McGraw & Wong, 1992; Vargha & Delaney, 2000; Fritz, Morris, & Richler, 2012; Han, 2019). Among the three optimised feature sets of sentiment (95), semantic (104), structural (13) features, we retained the top 17 features which had p values smaller than 0.001 and effect sizes larger than 0.1 as shown in Table 4.7.

The retained features were A15 (abstract terms relating to (the level) of safety/danger) ($p<0.001$, $\eta^2=0.22$), Affil_GI (words of affiliation or supportiveness) ($p<0.001$, $\eta^2=0.18$), wordy items ($p<0.001$, $\eta^2=0.16$), number of complex (3+ syllable) words ($p<0.001$, $\eta^2=0.16$), Intrj_GI (casual, slang words of agreement or disagreement) ($p<0.001$, $\eta^2=0.16$), Nonadlt_GI (words referring to infants through adolescents) ($p<0.001$, $\eta^2=0.14$), number of unique complex words of three syllables or more ($p<0.001$, $\eta^2=0.15$), misspelling (difficult words) ($p<0.001$, $\eta^2=0.15$), Sv_GI (verbs of mental, emotional states) ($p<0.001$, $\eta^2=0.15$), overused words ($p<0.001$, $\eta^2=0.14$), Hostile_GI (attitudes of hostility, aggressiveness) ($p<0.001$, $\eta^2=0.14$), happiness_GALC (words of happiness) ($p<0.001$, $\eta^2=0.13$), Z99 (difficult,

Table 4.7 *Mann Whitney U Test of the full dataset*

Test Statistics	Mann-Whitney U	Z	P (2-tailed)	Effect Size (η2)	Mean Parents	Mean Public
A15	311852.00	−22.99	0.00	0.22	2.58	9.83
Affil_GI	345476.00	−20.63	0.00	0.18	0.06	0.04
Wordy items	361566.50	−19.66	0.00	0.16	14.15	35.36
Number of complex (3+ syllable) words	361623.50	−19.65	0.00	0.16	93.80	206.71
Intrj_GI	364943.50	−19.45	0.00	0.16	0.014	0.009
Nonadlt_GI	387380.50	−18.46	0.00	0.14	0.012	0.003
Number of unique 3+ syllable words	369257.00	−19.19	0.00	0.15	59.10	113.40
Misspellings (difficult words)	374975.00	−19.00	0.00	0.15	4.15	20.83
Sv_GI	375847.00	−18.79	0.00	0.15	0.08	0.06
Overused words	382720.00	−18.39	0.00	0.14	12.26	27.51
Hostile_GI	384679.50	−18.26	0.00	0.14	0.04	0.03
Happiness_GALC	422401.00	−17.66	0.00	0.13	0.002	0.000
Z99 (difficult, out-of-dictionary words)	401235.50	−17.26	0.00	0.12	25.87	63.64
G1	480759.00	−15.80	0.00	0.10	0.32	1.38
Vice_GI	420847.50	−16.07	0.00	0.11	0.03	0.04
Z3	428935.50	−16.44	0.00	0.11	1.51	5.29
Role_GI	415833.50	−16.37	0.00	0.11	0.03	0.02

out-of-dictionary words) ($p<0.001$, $\eta^2=0.12$), G1 (terms relating to government, governmental activities) ($p<0.001$, $\eta^2=0.10$), Vice_GI (assessment of moral disapproval or misfortune) ($p<0.001$, $\eta^2=0.11$), Z3 (proper names) ($p<0.001$, $\eta^2=0.11$), Role_GI (identifiable, standardised individual human behaviour patterns, as used by sociologists) ($p<0.001$, $\eta^2=0.11$)).

Word classes in parentheses are those with statistically higher means in each sub-corpus and are from the three annotation systems: SEANCE, USAS, and Readability Studio.

Table 4.8 shows that features with statistically higher means in public-oriented environmental health information are consistent with a language style that is analytical, formal, complex, emphatic, and focuses on social responsibility. Conversely, features with statistically higher means in parent-oriented environmental health were associated with a highly supportive, informal, emotional, and interactive language style focusing on giving concrete instructions and advice. Among the top ranked linguistic features with the largest effect sizes (η^2), very few were related to the semantic content of the environmental health materials. As a result, the contents of the two large sets of environmental health texts collected did not differ significantly. Rather, the corpus analysis distinguished the two sets of corpus texts by identifying different stylistic features or different communicative styles. Materials developed for a general audience

Table 4.8 *A framework for the automatic evaluation of environmental health information user suitability*

Public-oriented communicative style		Parent-oriented communicative style	
Analytical	Higher ('A15')	**Supportive**	Higher ('Affil_GI')
Formal	Higher ('wordy items', 'G1', 'Z3')	**Informal**	Higher ('Intrj_GI')
Moral, ethical	Higher (Vice_GI)	**Emotional**	Higher ('Sv_GI' 'Hostile_GI' 'Happiness_GALC')
Emphatic	Higher ('overused words')	**Interactive**	Higher ('Nonadlt_GI')
Complex	Higher ('number of complex words, 'numbers of unique complex words', 'misspelling', 'Z99')	**Instructive**	Higher ('Role_GI')

communicate environmental health risks in a matter-of-fact style with limited emotional interaction. By contrast, resources developed for parents of young children demonstrated higher levels of emotional attachment and support, and a clear focus on engagement, instruction, and connection. It should be noted that the five dimensions of public-oriented communication style, i.e., analytical tone, formality, moral concern, lexical complexity, and emphasis, are highly interrelated. Together, they indicate a higher-level, less engaging communication style that is more suitable for mass communication. It has been demonstrated that the five dimensions of the parent-oriented communicative style – supportiveness, informality, emotional connections, instructiveness, and interactivity – are also compatible among these dimensions, as the intended audience for environmental health information is parents of young children. Table 4.8 provides a theoretical framework for evaluating the suitability of environmental health resources for different readers. The framework is data-driven and focused on health communicative style. It differs from current evaluation tools for written health materials such as widely used readability tools. Lexical complexity, which forms the basis for readability tools, is a component of this communicative style framework. Furthermore, this new framework highlights important new dimensions of effective communication, such as engagement and interaction, which are not included in current health information quality assessment guidelines.

As a result of examining the analytical framework developed using automatic feature optimisation, statistical ranking, and selection, four features which overlapped (Overused words, Z99, Z3, Role_GI) were removed and were replaced with three new ones (You_GI, Fear_EmoLex, Compare_GI) which focused on emotional, cognitive, and personal interaction of the environmental health texts with the intended readers. Two main objectives motivated this refinement process. First, to further improve the prediction accuracy of the new model. A second goal was to make the framework more linguistically interpretable so that the automatic evaluation can be more helpful in developing and evaluating environmental health education resources. Table 4.9 shows the comparison of the performance between the automatically developed (EF17) and the linguistically refined (RF16) models. It shows that the linguistically refined model (RF16) achieved on the testing data higher overall prediction accuracy (AUC: 0.940) compared to the automatically developed model (EF17) (AUC: 0.920), higher sensitivity (0.912) and higher specificity (0.866). Using z-score feature normalisation, the performance of the linguistically refined model based on the automatically developed model (EF17) was improved in terms of sensitivity

Table 4.9 *Performance of LR classifiers with effective and refined feature*

	Training data		Testing data				
LR	AUC Mean	SD.	AUC	Accuracy	Sensitivity	Specificity	Macro-F1
EF17	0.922	0.014	0.920	0.863	0.889	0.823	0.857
EF17 MM	0.931	0.009	0.930	0.872	0.885	0.852	0.866
EF17 L2	0.828	0.034	0.825	0.756	0.767	0.739	0.748
EF17 z-score	0.930	0.010	0.928	0.876	0.887	0.859	0.871
RF16	0.941	0.011	0.940	0.894	0.912	0.866	0.889
RF16 MM	0.944	0.010	0.947	0.900	0.903	0.894	0.896
RF16 L2	0.836	0.031	0.823	0.755	0.760	0.746	0.748
RF16 z-score	**0.944**	**0.010**	**0.947**	**0.904**	**0.908**	**0.898**	**0.900**

(0.908) and specificity (0.898). Using the paired sample t test, we will compare the performance of the final model (RF16) with other competing models to assess any statistically significant differences in sensitivity and specificity.

Next, we compared the area under the curve of the receiver operating characteristic (AUC of ROC) of the best model RF16 with other high performing, competing models emerged during the feature optimisation process. We selected some of the models with the highest AUC including All418 with z-score normalisation (with all three sets of original features; semantic: 115, sentiment: 270, structural: 33) (AUC: 0.979); All65 (joint optimisation of three sets of original features; semantic: 45, sentiment: 2, structural: 18) (AUC: 0.954); SUS212 with min-max normalisation (with three sets of individually optimised features; semantic: 104, sentiment: 95, structural: 13) (AUC: 0.977); EF17 with z-score normalisation (topic seventeen features with the largest statistical effect sizes after automatic feature optimisation; sentiment: 8, semantic: 4, structural: 5) (AUC: 0.928). RF16 with z-score normalisation had an AUC of 0.947 which was slightly lower than All418, All65, SUS212 MM models. The advantage of RF16 consists in its parsimony and efficiency with as little as sixteen features. RF16 is thus more informative for the development of linguistically interpretable models that can be implemented in the automatic assessment of the suitability of environmental health information for the intended readers, i.e., parents versus the public.

4.6 Communicative Style Matters for Environmental Health Communication

The performance evaluation of various competing machine learning models identified the best analytical model. It is the most parsimonious model with as few as sixteen linguistic features but very high performance in terms of overall classification accuracy, and high precision rates to predict binary outcomes, i.e., materials suitable for environmental health education of parents of young children versus those more suitable for public communication purposes. A multiple logistic regression model was fit to interpret these features as predictors to forecast the likelihood of a certain environmental health text being suitable for parental environmental health education or not. Table 4.10 shows the results of the multiple logistic regression analysis. All linguistic features were standardised using z-score transformation to increase their normality for multiple logistic regression.

Table 4.10 *Multiple logistic regression (enter) of refined, standardised sixteen features*

Features	Standardised Coefficient Beta	S.D.	S.E.	Wald	Sig.	EXP(B)	95% C.I. for EXP(B)		Z scores
							Lower	Upper	
Types of multi-syllable words	1.91	67.43	0.39	23.81	0.00	6.73	3.13	14.47	4.88
Abstract terms of safety/danger	−1.11	9.19	0.15	53.11	0.00	0.33	0.24	0.44	−7.29
Verbose expressions	−1.30	29.9	0.24	29.92	0.00	0.27	0.17	0.43	−5.47
Terms relating to government and governmental activities	−0.52	2.23	0.11	21.54	0.00	0.59	0.47	0.74	−4.64
Casual, slang words of dis/agreement	0.48	0.069	0.08	32.77	0.00	1.62	1.37	1.91	5.72
Words referring to infants/adolescents	0.94	0.011	0.11	74.16	0.00	2.55	2.06	3.16	8.61
Verbs of mental or emotional states	0.51	0.021	0.09	34.42	0.00	1.66	1.40	1.97	5.87
Words of affiliation or supportiveness	0.51	0.021	0.09	35.02	0.00	1.67	1.41	1.98	5.92
Words of happiness	0.85	0.002	0.13	44.01	0.00	2.34	1.82	3.00	6.63
Attitudes of hostility or aggressiveness	0.72	0.019	0.08	73.27	0.00	2.05	1.74	2.41	8.56
Assessment of moral disapproval	−0.61	0.018	0.08	54.67	0.00	0.54	0.46	0.64	−7.39
Tokens of multi-syllable words	−1.14	152.2	0.45	6.29	0.01	0.32	0.13	0.78	−2.51
Difficult words	−1.43	26.11	0.20	53.26	0.00	0.24	0.16	0.35	−7.30
Second person pronouns	−0.88	0.02	0.08	130.99	0.00	0.42	0.36	0.48	−11.45
Emotions of fear	−0.60	0.026	0.09	46.62	0.00	0.55	0.46	0.65	−6.83
Words of comparison	−0.34	0.006	0.07	23.30	0.00	0.71	0.62	0.82	−4.83

Table 4.10 shows that fifteen of the sixteen features were statistically significant predictors (p smaller than 0.001) of the binary outcomes. Since all the original features were standardised, the interpretation of standardised coefficient beta is that with the increase of one standard deviation of the predictor feature, the log odds of a health text being suitable for parental environmental education will increase by a standardised coefficient beta. Positive, statistically significant coefficients are indicative of predictors of environmental health texts suitable for parental education purposes, whereas negative, statistically significant coefficients are indicatives of linguistic features as predictors for environmental health texts being suitable for public communication use. The column Exp(B) is the odds ratio between parent-oriented versus public-oriented environmental health texts. Odds ratios are obtained by taking the exponential of log odds or coefficients. Odds ratios larger than one suggest higher probabilities for texts to be suitable for parental environmental health education, whereas odds ratios lower than one suggest the opposite, i.e., higher probabilities for texts to be suitable for public communication. For example, with an increase of 1 standard deviation (sixty-seven words) of unique complex words (with three or more syllables), the log-odds and odds of the text being suitable for parental environmental health education increase by 1.91 and 673 per cent, respectively. For A15 (abstract terms relating to the level of safety/danger), with the increase of 1 standard deviation (nine words), the log-odds and odds for the text being suitable for parental environmental education decrease by 1.11 and 67 per cent, respectively. For G1 (terms relating to government and governmental activities), with the increase of 1 standard deviation (two words), the log-odds and odds of the text being suitable for parental environmental education decrease by 0.52 and 41 per cent. The three newly added features are shown at the bottom of Table 4.10, For You_GI (second person pronouns like you, yourself, yourselves), with the increase of 1 standard deviation (0.03 words), the log-odds and odds for the text being suitable for parental environmental health education reduces by 0.88 and 58 per cent. For Fear_EmoLex (emotions of fear, negative emotions), with the increase of 1 standard deviation (0.02 words) the log-odds and odds for the text being suitable for parental environmental education reduces by 0.6 and 45 per cent. For Compare_GI (words of comparison), with the increase of 1 standard deviation (0.006 words) the log-odds and odds for the text being suitable for parental environmental education reduces by 0.34 and 29 per cent.

To better understand the relationship between predictor characteristics and assessment outcomes, we plotted the forest plot of multivariable

Table 4.11 *Refined framework for the automated evaluation of environmental health information suitability*

Public-oriented communicative style		Parent-oriented communicative style	
Analytical	Higher ('A15', Compare_GI)	**Supportive**	Higher ('Affil_GI')
Formal	Higher ('wordy items', 'G1')	**Informal**	Higher ('Intrj_GI')
Moral, Ethical	Higher (Vice_GI, Fear_EmoLex)	**Emotional**	Higher ('Sv_GI' 'Hostile_GI' 'Happiness_GALC')
Interactive	Higher ('You_GI')	**Interactive**	Higher ('Nonadlt_GI')
Complex	Higher ('number of complex words', 'misspelling')	**Complex**	Higher ('numbers of unique complex words')

logistic regression on a logarithmic scale as shown in Figure 4.2. On the forest plot, the list of features on the left are interpretations of the original annotation categories shown in Appendix 4.1. The right-hand side shows the odds ratios and confidence intervals for each linguistic class. The middle line represents the odds ratio of one. The squares on either side of the middle line represent the significance levels for each linguistic category. The significance levels were set at ${}^{a}p < .001$. ${}^{b}p < .01$. ${}^{c}p < .05$. The lower the significance level, the more significant a linguistic feature is as a predictor in a multivariable logistic regression equation. Features with squares to the left of the middle line are statistically significant predictors of being suitable for general environmental health communication, and features with squares to the right of the middle line are significant predictors of being relevant, suitable for parental environmental health education. We updated the framework for the automatic evaluation of the suitability of environmental health information for different audiences based on the distribution of predictor features (Table 4.8). The updated version was presented in Table 4.11.

The updated automated evaluation framework is similar to the initial model (Table 4.8) developed through automatic feature selection. First, the language of environmental health information for the general public was more analytical. Two linguistic features emerged as statistically significant predictors of the relevance of texts for public-oriented environmental communication: A15 (abstract terms relating to the level of safety/danger)

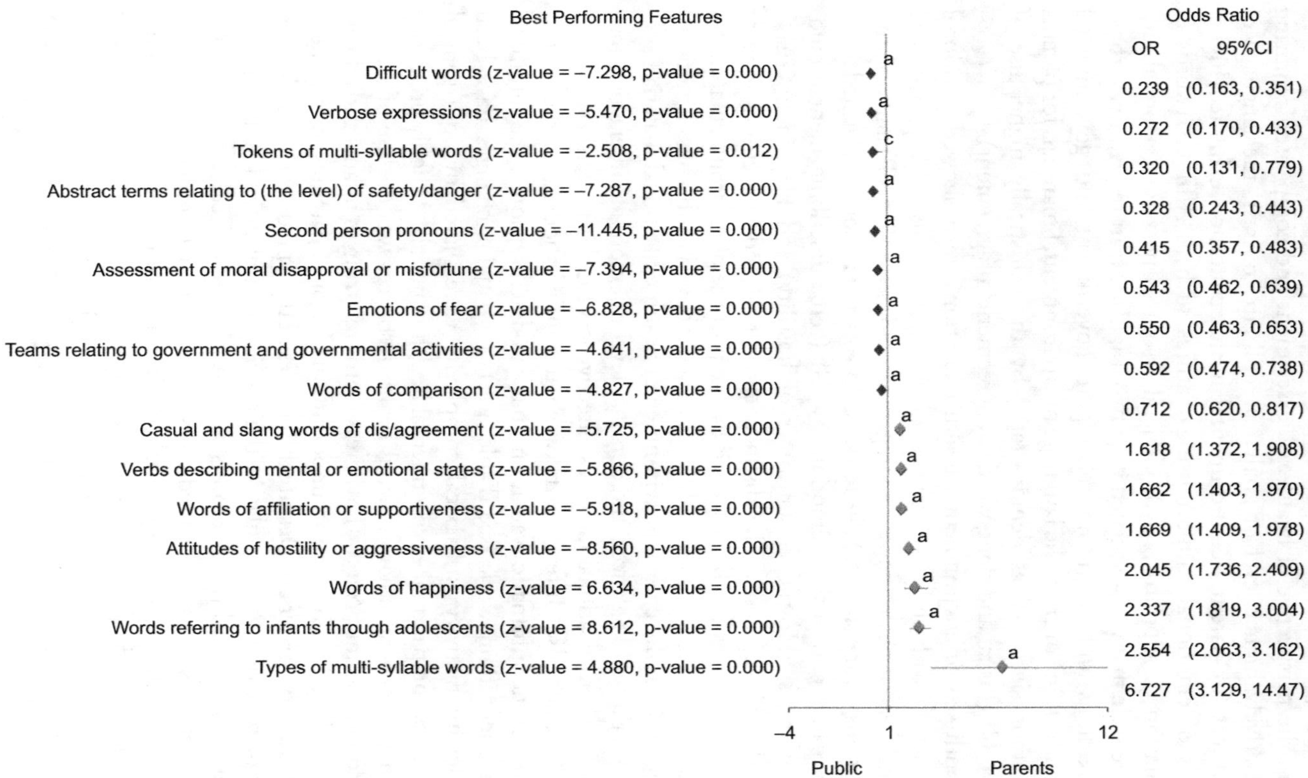

Figure 4.2 Forest plot of multivariable logistic regression.
[a] $p < .001$. [b] $p < .01$. [c] $p < .05$. The x-axis is a logarithmic, not linear scale.

and Compare_GI (words of comparison). Both factors suggest that general resources provided an analysis of environmental health events and issues from the perspective of health risk assessment and comparison requiring a relatively higher level of analytical skill. In contrast, the language of resources for parental environmental health education exhibited higher levels of emotional support using features such as Affil_GI (words of affiliation or supportiveness). General resources possessed a formal language style that was associated with two linguistic features: wordy, verbose expressions and G1 (terms relating to government and governmental activities). In contrast, the language of environmental materials for parents was more informal as demonstrated by the statistically higher use of Intrj_GI (casual and slang words of agreement/disagreement).

Both sets of environmental health educational texts showed emotional interaction with the target audiences. An increased use of expressions of moral disapproval was observed in general resources (Vice_GI) and negative emotions (Fear_EmoLex) like fears. Parent-oriented resources featured a mix of negative and positive emotions Sv_GI (verbs describing mental, emotional states), Hostile_GI (attitudes of hostility) and Happiness_GALC (words of happiness). The distinctively critical and concerning tone of general resources can be explained by the purpose of environmental health communications: to raise public awareness about health risks. Emotional interaction in the parental environmental health educational materials suggest that a more balanced and personal level of emotional interaction may increase the educational materials' effectiveness for this readership.

There are also differences between the initial model and the refined model of the automatic evaluation. In the updated version of the automatic assessment framework (see Table 4.12), two major changes have been made: interactivity and lexical complexity were shared by both general resources and parental environmental health materials. A highly predictive feature of general environmental health resources was the use of second person pronouns (You_GI), whereas words referring to infants and adolescents (Nonadlt_GI) were an important predictor of parental environmental education materials. Despite differences in their predictor features, both sets of materials were similar in their lexical complexity. The number of complex words (three or more syllables) and the difficulty of the words were two of the strongest predictors for general environmental resources, while for parent-oriented materials, the number of unique (three or more syllables) complex words was the strongest indicator. Both general and parent-oriented environmental health materials were lexically complex, based on this finding. As a verification, we calculated the SMOG Index

Table 4.12 *Automatic assessment framework*

Dimensions	Public-oriented Communication	Parent-oriented Communication
Cognitive style	Analytical	Supportive, aptitude
Formality	Formal	Informal
Emotional interaction	Higher level, moral, ethical (Primarily negative)	Personal level (Mixed emotions, supportive)
Reference	You, yourselves	Children, boys, girls, teens
Lexical complexity	Higher	High

scores for both sets of texts. For public-oriented environmental texts, the mean SMOG score was 13 (SD: 2.09, S.E.0.067); for parent-oriented health materials, the mean SMOG score was 11 (SD: 1.64, S.E.0.044). Accordingly, general resources need minimal college education as opposed to parental education materials that require year 11 or higher education, and both levels are significantly higher than the recommended reading level of the WHO, which is grade 8. This finding helps to explain why binary classifiers developed using scores of readability tools (Flesch Reading Ease Index, Gunning Fog Index, SMOG Index) are not very accurate. Similarly, this indicates that information relevance or suitability is a much more complex concept than the traditional measure of readability based solely on lexical complexity. This automatic assessment framework identified the following five large dimensions that are useful in assessing and predicting the suitability of environmental health materials for different audiences: cognitive style (analytic for general materials; supportive for parental materials), formality (formal for general communication materials; informal for parental materials), emotional interaction (higher level, moral disapproval for general materials; personal level mixed emotions for parental materials), personal reference ('you' for general environmental materials; 'children, teenagers' for parental materials), and lexical complexity (polysyllabic words).

4.7 Conclusion

Due to climate change and the complexity of environmental health risks, environmental health communication and education has become an increasingly pressing research topic in recent years. The WHO has developed a new strategic framework for effective health communications that stresses the importance of tailoring health messages for different audiences. The purpose of this chapter was to translate the WHO guidelines and policies into empirical research tools and instruments to facilitate the development and evaluation of environmental health information for targeted audiences. Readability formulas have been the standard method of assessing the readability of health materials for many decades. There has been criticism of the ineffectiveness of these tools by health authorities such as the Agency for Healthcare Research and Quality and the U.S. Department of Health and Human Services when assessing the suitability of health information for different readers. Therefore, the goal of our study was to develop a linguistically enhanced framework for evaluating the usefulness of environmental health information for parental education in comparison with resources developed for public communication.

This chapter faced two major challenges: first, there was no theoretical linguistic framework based on which to develop automated evaluation systems; second, in previous studies, the relevance of certain linguistic features for effective health communication has been touched upon, but it remains unknown whether those features significantly, marginally, or at all improve the performance of machine learning models to assess the suitability of texts of environmental communication for different readers. As such, qualitative and quantitative approaches were distinctively parallel in the current evaluation of environmental health information. In order to address these challenges, we combined automatic feature optimisation with statistical ranking of optimised features based on their effect sizes before developing an interpretable, descriptive model for the computerised evaluation of environmental health resources for parents versus the general public.

There are advantages to this new method of evaluating environmental health information. First, by integrating quantitative and qualitative approaches, the computerised evaluation process has achieved evaluation cost-effectiveness and ensured the results are both interpretable and informative. Machine learning models with complex parameters often have less interpretable results, which are ineffective for revising and adjusting the linguistic features of health materials to increase their suitability for target audiences. The new model developed, however, can easily identify linguistic features that are statistically significant predictors of whether a text is suitable for parent education. Health resource developers can use this information to make targeted changes and amendments to less effective educational resources. In addition, it provides environmental health educators with a number of necessary assessment instruments.

The second advantage of our new model is its adaptability and flexibility. A logistic regression model predicts a text's suitability based on the likelihood that it belongs to a class. The default probability threshold is 0.5. The text assigned probabilities equal to or greater than 0.5 will be predicted as suitable for parental education purposes, while the text assigned probabilities less than 0.5 will be automatically classified as unsuitable for parental education. However, the default threshold is not fixed. It can be increased or lowered based on the research needs. Threshold adjustment directly impacts the accuracy of automated classification. For example, increasing the probability threshold increases model sensitivity and false positivity for parental education materials, if the research priority is to increase prediction accuracy in terms of model sensitivity, or text materials correctly predicted as suitable for parental education. We could lower the probability threshold if the goal of the research is to identify texts not suitable for parental education, which will result in a higher specificity and higher false negatives. Decisions about the probability threshold for predicting are often based on trade-offs. In this study, threshold probability of 0.5 represents the best trade-off, as this study sought to develop a balanced assessment model.

There are however limitations that warrant further research. Interviews could not be conducted to solicit feedback on the appropriateness of environmental health materials from the target users, parents of young children, and classify the feedback based on demographic characteristics such as educational level, cultural background, native language, and so on. This study assumed that the typical reader of parental environmental health educational resources online was a parent with a Year 10 education who came from an English-speaking background. This assumption has simplified the practical scenarios of environmental health education and communication in multicultural countries. To develop machine learning evaluation systems that can provide more personalised evaluation results for readers from diverse backgrounds, it is necessary to gather information from different reader groups and modify the automated evaluation tools to reflect their practical requirements for accessible, relevant, and effective environmental health educational information, which provides the focus of future research.

CHAPTER 5

Improving the Readability of Japanese Translations of Natural Disaster Risks Through Predictive Automated English Information Design

5.1 Cross-Lingual Communication of Natural Disasters

Unprecedented heatwaves, cyclones, floods, and bushfires are no longer rare events but are instead becoming the new normal (National Disaster Risk Information Services Capability (NDRISC), 2020). A key recommendation of the NDRISC report is that national capability needs to be developed urgently 'to assist users to access, use and interpret disaster information [through knowledge brokerage and translation]'. Natural events can have a disproportionate impact on people with limited access to disaster preparedness and risk reduction information (Villeneuve, 2021). In many cases it is a matter of life or death. People around the world have suffered and continue to suffer significant human and economic losses due to lack of disaster preparedness. Disaster losses are avoidable, but only when there are personal disaster preparedness, resilience, and knowledge (Gowan, Sloan, & Kirk, 2015). Accessible translation of disaster information is critical to support the public to develop disaster preparedness and resilience. However, currently, disaster information is not available in accessible formats for people who require translation assistance in multicultural countries (Nepal, Banerjee, Perry, & Scott, 2012; O'Brien, Federici, Cadwell, Marlowe, & Gerber, 2018; Ogie & Perez, 2020; Xiang, Gerber, & Zhang, 2021). Existing translation research tends to theorise and evluate the quality of translation in terms of linguistic accuracy and fluency (Nida, 1975; Venuti, 2017). Even though these generic principles can inform and guide standard translation practice, they have important methodological limitations in the context of health translation as literacy development tools (Sørensen & Brand, 2014). Translation for educational purposes requires tailoring the translation to increase its understandability, trustworthiness, and cultural affinity for the reader (Lin & Ji, 2019; Ji & Sørensen, & Bouillon, 2021). Translations of increased linguistic and cultural accessibility and inclusiveness can have significant impact on the knowledge and self-management of health risks among vulnerable communities such as multicultural people with limited education (Ji, Taibi, & Crezee, 2019; Murphy, Abdi, & Seale, 2020).

This chapter proposes a novel approach to the development and assessment of English disaster and environmental risk information for people from diverse language and cultural backgrounds who require readable, more accessible translations, regardless of education level, and cultural or linguistic background. To illustrate the development of machine learning classifiers for the purpose of the predictive assessment of the likelihood that an English text will be translated into an accessible language, we will use Japanese as an illustrative case study, given the language and cultural contrast between English and Japanese.

5.2 Sources of English Information on Natural Disaster Risks

Appendix 5.1 provides the list of online texts on disaster and environmental risks from emergency services and health authorities.

5.3 Linguistic Annotation of the English Source Texts

Tables 5.1 and 5.2 provide the statistics of the corpus created for developing machine learning models.

Feature annotation was done using Readability Studio (Oleander Software) and an automatic semantic annotation system (USAS) developed by the University of Lancaster in the UK. Readability Studio added twenty-seven natural language features regarding morphological, lexical and syntactic complexity of the texts: medical jargon, number of unique words, repeated words, article mismatches, wording errors, redundant phrases, overused words, wordy items, clichés, number of proper nouns, number of numerals, average number of characters, average number of syllables, number of monosyllabic words, number of unique monosyllabic words, number of complex (3+ syllable) words, number of unique 3+ syllable words, number of long (6+ characters) words, number of unique long words, average number of sentences per paragraph, number of difficult sentences (more than twenty-two words), average sentence length, passive voice, sentences that begin with conjunctions, number of interrogative sentences (questions), number of exclamatory sentences. USAS added twenty-two large semantic categories: general/abstract terms, medicine/Health, arts and culture, emotion, food, government, dwelling, employment, sports, living Things, locations, measurements,

Table 5.1 *Corpus statistics – ratio between Part of Speech (POS) categories and the total number of words in the corpus*

ADJ	ADP	ADV	AUX	CCONJ	DET	NOUN
Adjective	Ad-position	Adverb	Auxiliary	Coordinating conjunction	Determiner	Noun
0.085	0.117	0.029	0.066	0.051	0.084	0.282
NUM	PART	PRON	PROPN	PUNCT	SCONJ	VERB
Numeral	Particle	Pronoun	Proper Noun	Punctuation	Subordinating conjunction	Verb
0.013	0.027	0.05	0.054	0.122	0.018	0.129

Table 5.2 *Corpus statistics – lexical and textual complexity measures*

Total number of words	Average number of unique words	Average number of characters	Average number of syllables	Average number of monosyllabic words	Average number of unique monosyllabic words	Average Number of complex three-syllable words
88,678	0.866	5.057	1.685	0.586	0.481	0.183
Average number of unique three-syllable words	Average Number of long six-character words	Average number of unique long words	Average use of passive voice	Average number of punctuations	Average Sentiment Score	Average frequency in BNC
0.171	0.37	0.346	0.013	4.236	0.021	312

general substances, education, speech acts, social actions, time, environment, psychology, science/tech, names and grammar and out of dictionary words. We also used a large number of readability indexes to measure the linguistic complexity of the original English texts including Automated readability index (ARI), Bormuth Cloze Mean, Bormuth Grade Placement, Coleman-Liau (grade levels), Coleman-Liau (predicted Cloze scores), New Dale-Chall, Danielson-Bryan 1, Danielson-Bryan 2, Degrees of Reading Power, Degrees of Reading Power (GE), ELF, EFLAW, Flesch-Kincaid Index, Flesch Reading Ease Index, FORCAST, Fry, Gunning Fog Index, Harris-Jacobson Lix (index values), Lix (grade levels), Modified SMOG, New ARI, SARI, New Fog Count, PSK Dale-Chall, Rix (index values), Rix (grade levels), SMOG, Spache Revised and Wheeler-Smith.

5.4 Assessment of Japanese Readability (the Japanese Text Readability Measurement Scale)

We used the Japanese Text Readability Measurement Scale (JTRMS) developed by Jaeho Lee at Waseda University, Japan (Hasebe, Lee, & Bekeš, 2019). The system classifies the input text into one of the following six levels as shown in Table 5.3. In our study, we used a conservative score, 2.5 as the threshold to define the accessibility of the Japanese translations of English disaster information. That is, we classified Japanese translations as readable translations if their JTRMS scores were higher than 2.5, and classified the translations as non-readable if their JTRMS scores were equal or below 2.5.

Appendix 5.2 provides examples of Japanese texts within different readability ranges.

5.5 Linguistic Feature Selection for Developing Machine Learning Classifiers

Figure 5.1 and Table 5.4 show the result of the logistic regression analysis of the impact of six linguistic features of the English texts on the readability of the Japanese translations. It shows that increasing the use of two linguistic features in the English source texts can significantly reduce the complexity of Japanese translations: punctuation (PUNCT) (O.R. 0.000153, 95 per cent confidence interval, C.I. 0.000033, 0.001, $p<0.001$), and proper nouns (PROPN) (O.R. 0.000393, 95 per cent C.I. 0.000098, 0.002, $p<0.001$). By contrast, increasing the use of ad-positions (ADP) in the English texts, the complexity of their Japanese translations will increase significantly (O.R. 12.537, 95 per cent

Table 5.3 *Grading system of the Japanese Text Readability Measurement Scale (JTRMS)*

Level	Score Range	Description
Lower-Elementary (Very easy)	5.5–6.4	Can understand basic Japanese expressions, especially simple sentences. Cannot understand complex sentence structures such as compound sentences and serial modifier structures.
Upper-Elementary (Easy)	4.5–5.4	Can understand basic vocabulary and grammatical items. Can understand basic compound sentences using the -te form, etc.
Lower-Intermediate (So-so)	3.5–4.4	Comprehension of relatively plain text, and the ability to grasp the content of even somewhat incoherent texts.
Upper-intermediate (Slightly difficult)	2.5–3.4	Able to comprehend the general content of somewhat specialised texts and can comprehend texts at the level of daily life with little difficulty.
Lower-Advanced (Difficult)	1.5–2.4	Can understand most specialised texts. Can understand complex structures found in literary and other works.
Upper-Advanced (Very difficult)	0.5–1.4	Can understand highly technical texts without difficulty. Has no difficulty with any Japanese text.

C.I. 2.001, 78.546, $p=0.007$). Ad-position refers to prepositions and postpositions such as in, under, towards, before, which are used to indicate the relationships between nouns within a sentence, adding to the complexity of translation to a distinct language such as Japanese. Higher scores of the original English texts on three readability indexes also proved significant predictors of the complexity of their Japanese translations: Flesch-Kincaid Index (O.R. 1.149, 95 per cent C.I. 1.086, 1.217, $p<0.001$), Danielson-Byran 1 (O.R.3.416, 95 per cent C.I. 2.593, 4.5, $p<0.001$), and Coleman-Liau estimated cloze scores (O.R. 1.058, 95 per cent C.I.1.042, 1.074, $p<0.001$).

5.6 Comparing Machine Learning Classifiers

Figure 5.2 and Table 5.5 compare the performance of the machine learning classifiers developed on the testing dataset: linear support vector machine (SVM) and radial basis function kernel (RBF) SVM with six linguistic features and three different transformation methods, i.e., z-score (ZSN), min-max normalisation (MMN), and logarithmic normalisation (L2 N).

Table 5.4 *Logistic regression analysis of the impact on English linguistic features on Japanese translations' readability*

							95% C.I. for EXP(B)		
English Linguistic Features	B *	S.E.	Wald	df	Sig.	Exp(B)	Lower	Upper	z-scores
ADP	2.529	0.936	7.295	1	0.007	12.537	2.001	78.546	2.702
PUNCT	−11.039	1.007	120.203	1	<.001	0.000153	0.000033	0.001	−10.962
PROPN	−7.841	0.707	122.861	1	<.001	0.000393	0.000098	0.002	−11.091
Flesch-Kincaid	0.139	0.029	23.09	1	<.001	1.149	1.086	1.217	4.793
Danielson-Bryan 1	1.228	0.141	76.313	1	<.001	3.416	2.593	4.5	8.709
Coleman-Liau (pred. cloze scores)	0.056	0.008	51.702	1	<.001	1.058	1.042	1.074	7

*The predicted membership is Japanese translations below the readability threshold of 2.5.

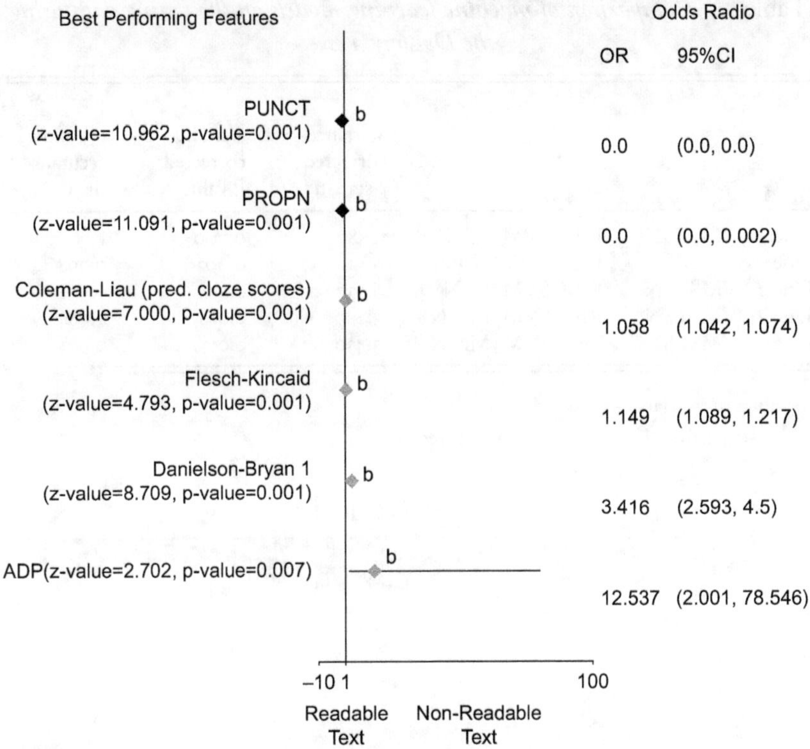

Figure 5.1 Logistic regression forest plot (a: $p<0.001$, b: $p<0.01$, c: $p<0.05$).

The result shows that in terms of the size of the area under the curve of the receiver operating characteristic (ROC), linear SVM with z-score normalisation (Linear_SVM_ZSN) (AUC=0.862) outperformed all other machine learning classifiers with the same set of English linguistic features: RBF_SVM_ZSN (AUC=0.856) ($p<0.001$), Linear_SVM_L2 N (AUC=0.770, $p=0.002$), RBF_SVM_L2 N (AUC=0.776, $p=0.002$), RBF_SVM_MMN (AUC=0.852, $p=0.016$), and Linear_SVM_MMN (AUC=0.855, $p=0.013$).

Figure 5.3 shows that 75 per cent of English text associated with readable translations was assigned a probability under 51 per cent, and 80 per cent of English text associated with non-readable translations was assigned a probability equal or larger than 50 per cent.

Table 5.5 *Comparison of machine learning models on the testing data using the DeLong Test*

I	j	Variance-corrected t-statistic	Variance-corrected P value *	Probability of i more accurate than j **
Linear SVM_ZSN	RBF_SVM_ZSN	11.587	0.000	1
Linear SVM_ZSN	Linear SVM_L2 N	6.121	0.002	0.998
Linear SVM_ZSN	RBF_SVM_L2 N	6.237	0.002	0.998
Linear SVM_ZSN	RBF_SVM_MMN	3.247	0.016	0.984
Linear SVM_ZSN	Liner SVM_MMN	3.430	0.013	0.987

*p values are variance-corrected

**Bayesian estimation of the comparison result.

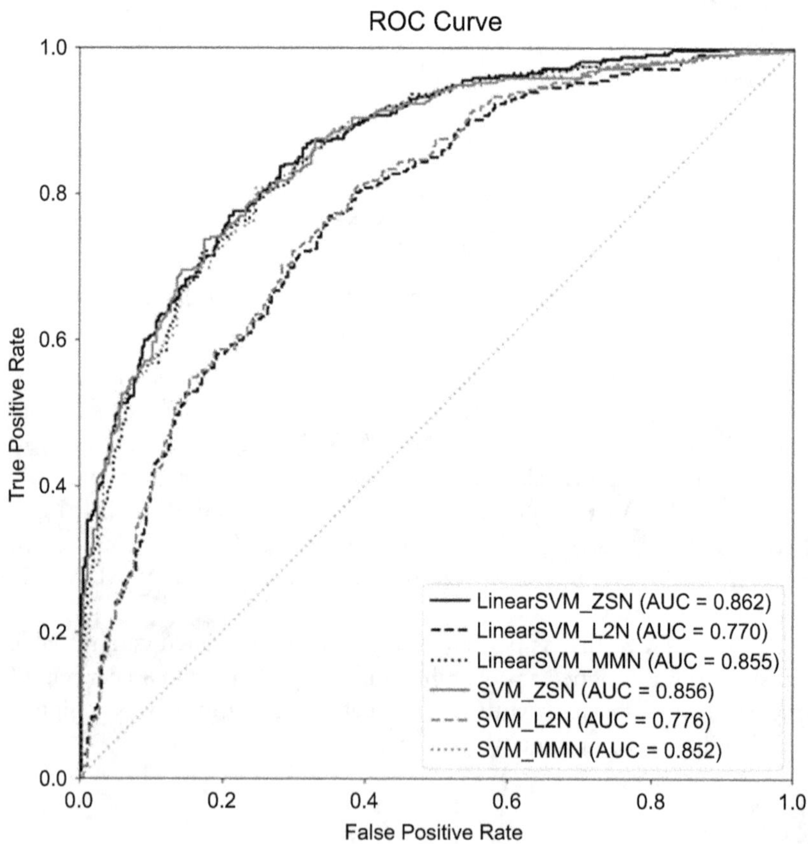

Figure 5.2 Area under the curve of the receiver operating characteristic (ROC) of the models on the testing dataset.

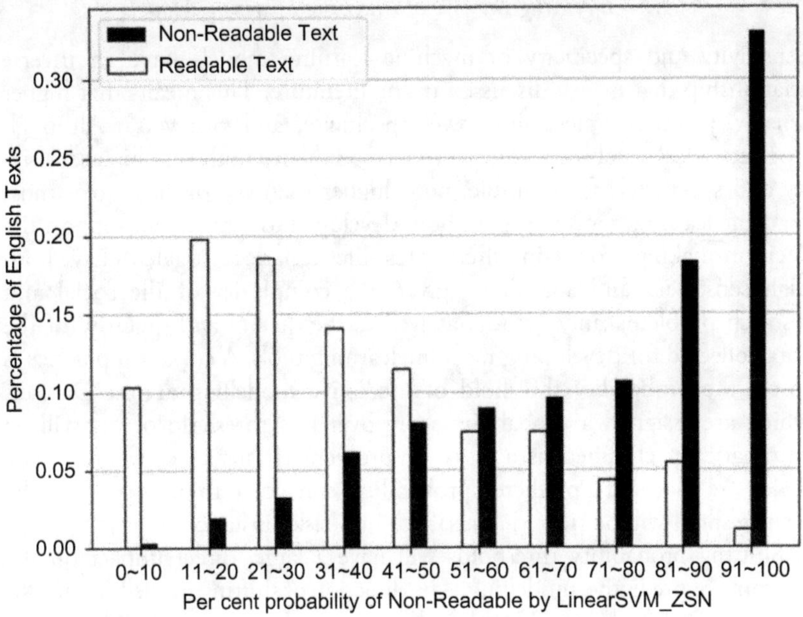

Figure 5.3 Percentage of English texts associated with readable or non-readable Japanese translations assigned by the best performing SVM classifier with six English linguistic features (Linear SVM_6) to each 10 per cent probability bin.

5.7 Setting Thresholds of Sensitivity and Specificity Pairs of Machine Learning Models

For a certain machine learning model, the size of its area under the curve (AUC) or overall accuracy is fixed. However, higher AUC or model accuracy does not necessarily translate into the practical usefulness of the model in the clinic or the health research context. The selection of probability thresholds, which are the values used to define the presence or absence of a certain outcome, can have an important impact on the usefulness of the model. In this section, we will explain the selection of the best probability threshold for the best-performing SVM to maximise the practical utility of the model developed for the purpose of predicting and reducing the risk of English natural disaster information being translated into written Japanese of lower readability, comprehensibility, and public accessibility.

5.7.1 *Deciding the Use of Machine Learning Models*

Sensitivity and specificity of machine learning models have an inverse relationship that is well discussed in the literature. This means that higher sensitivity often comes with lower specificity, and vice versa. Although a perfect, ideal machine learning model would have both very high sensitivity and specificity, for example, both higher than 0.9 or close to 1, most machine learning tools that have been developed to inform and support the decision-making process in different real-life scenarios struggle to have both high sensitivity and specificity, given the complexity of the social and research problems under study, as well as the quality and quantity of the data collected for developing machine learning tools. A common practice is to set the probability threshold of predictive modelling at 0.5. Datasets which are assigned a probability score over this threshold of 0.5 will be automatically classified as a risky or problematic instance, whereas data which are allocated a predicted probability score equal to or lower than the 0.5 threshold will be treated as a safe or non-risky instance.

Shifting probability thresholds will have a large, direct impact on the outcome of predictive modelling. The direction of shifting modelling thresholds also needs to be considered in the context of the purpose and practical utility of the model. Machine learning models of higher sensitivity and often lower specificity lend themselves well for ruling out textual samples or data that are considered 'risky' or of concern. In our study, this kind of data refers to textual excerpts of English disaster information which are more likely to be translated to Japanese of lower readability or accessibility to the Japanese public. The reason is that machine learning models of higher sensitivity have lower probability thresholds. As a result, if an English textual sample is assigned a predicted probability score lower than the predefined threshold, its odds of being translated to written Japanese of lower readability will be low and can thus be ruled out as an instance requiring further revision and adjustment to improve its translatability into more readable, accessible written Japanese. By contrast, machine learning models of higher specificity, and consequently lower sensitivity, are suitable and useful for ruling in risky or 'of concern' data that require further improvement. That is because higher specificity is the result of raising the probability threshold of a machine learning model. In our study, with increased probability thresholds, if a certain English textual sample is predicted to be 'risky' or less translatable into accessible, readable Japanese, its odds of generating a problematic Japanese translation will be higher, and such instances of English texts are thus ruled out.

The question here is to select a probability cutoff that can maximise the practical usefulness of an often imperfect, real machine learning model, given its fixed AUC or accuracy, often ranging between 0.7 and 0.8 that is indicative of a working model. When deciding on courses of action following the predictive modelling outcome, we need to know the likelihood or odds of a risky event after the assessment, also known as the posterior probability of the event. For example, in our study, the result of the machine learning prediction can be interpreted as the probability or likelihood of an English source text leading to a Japanese translation of a readability level that is lower than that of the predefined probability threshold, after we have applied the predictive modelling. Posterior probability should differ from the prior probability of an event, which represents our existing knowledge before using the machine learning tools to update and correct our understanding of the prevalence of that risky event.

The result of the machine learning provides a predictive assessment which indicates whether the English source text is likely to be translated into more readable and accessible Japanese, the posterior probability is calculated by multiplying the prior probability with the negative likelihood ratio (LR-) of the model, which is often lower than the prior probability. By contrast, if the modelling result indicates that the English source text is likely to cause readability issues of its Japanese translations, the posterior probability is computed by multiplying the prior probability with the positive likelihood ratio (LR+) of the model, which is higher than the prior probability.

In making decisions over whether actions are needed to reduce the predicted risks of a certain risky event or undesirable outcome, a common practice is to set the positive likelihood ratio (LR+) at 5 or higher. A LR+ of 5 means that the posterior odds of a risky event or outcome, based on the assessment, will be five times the prior probability, justifying and supporting the decision to take actions to avoid the occurrence of risky events over inaction. The higher the LR+, the stronger the evidence to support the decision to intervene. By contrast, if the purpose of the predictive modelling is to rule out instances of risky or harmful nature, or to identify instances of safe and desirable outcomes, we can use the negative likelihood ratio (LR-) to compute the posterior likelihood of the risky event. Similar to the utilisation of the positive likelihood ratio (LR+) function of predictive modelling, to justify decisions of inaction or not to intervene, for example, revision of the English source text to improve the readability of its Japanese translation, the posterior probability needs to be small enough when compared to the prior probability of the event. A common practice is to set the LR- at 0.2 or below. A LR- of 0.2 translates into a posterior probability that is 80 per cent lower than the prior probability. In more stringent scenarios such as the predictive assessment of harmful outcomes in the clinic, an acceptable LR+ and LR- can be set at 10 and 0.1, respectively to best support decision making with strong evidence.

As discussed earlier, the practical utility of machine learning models largely depends on the selection of the probability threshold which subsequently affects the sensitivity and specificity of the predictive modelling. To maximise the practical usefulness of the modelling tool, we often select machine learning models of positive likelihood ratios (LR+) higher than 5 and negative likelihood ratios (LR-) lower than 0.2.

Computation of likelihood ratios is based on the sensitivity and specificity of the model as follows:

$$\mathbf{LR+} = \mathbf{sensitivity} \ / \ \mathbf{1 - specificity}$$
$$\mathbf{LR-} = \mathbf{1 - sensitivity} \ / \ \mathbf{specificity}$$

Having selected the desired or practically useful positive and negative likelihood ratios (LR+ =5, LR- = 0.2), it becomes easier to identify the best, and most informative probability cutoff of a predictive modelling tool, and the sensitivity and specificity pair associated with the selected probability threshold along the receiver operating characteristic curve (ROC), representing the overall performance of the modelling.

The next practical question to consider is the main function of the machine learning model developed, that is, to support the targeted, cost-effective improvement of the translatability of English disaster information to Japanese, or to simply detect instances of English texts that are at higher risks of generating less readable and accessible Japanese translations. If the main function of the predictive tool is the former, higher sensitivity and lower negative likelihood ratios (LR- < = 0.2) are more desirable. If the purpose of the machine learning model developed is the latter, that is, detection of highly risky or less translatable English texts, higher specificity, and higher positive likelihood ratios (LR> =5) are more useful. Despite that predictive modelling has been extensively used for the purpose of risk detection and monitoring, in our study, we decide to leverage this research technique to improve the cost-effectiveness, efficiency of designing English disaster information that is of higher translatability, accessibility in a distinct language and cultural environment, using Japanese as an example to illustrate the automated predictive assessment process that can be replicated with other languages, especially under-resourced and minority languages to help reduce persistent inequality in accessing English natural disaster information among vulnerable communities in a changing global climate and environment.

In this chapter, the main function of the machine learning models developed is their ability to predict with high precision, the likelihood that English disaster information will be translated into Japanese which is at an acceptable level of readability or not. To be more specific, the two practical utilities of the machine learning classifiers developed are first, the model's ability to predict the likelihood of translations of low readability (equal or under the threshold), and second, the model's ability to predict the likelihood of translations of high readability (larger than the threshold).

Theoretically, the performance of machine learning models is assessed by model sensitivity and specificity. The relationship between sensitivity and specificity is inverse, which means that with the increase in sensitivity, i.e., the ability of machine learning models to detect positive cases or Japanese translations of low readability, specificity, or a model's ability to detect negative cases or Japanese translations of high readability and accessibility will decrease, and vice versa. Therefore, the model accuracy, or the average value of model sensitivity and specificity provides a balanced indicator of the model's overall performance. The table (Table 5.6) shows that the model balanced accuracy is the highest, 0.78 when the threshold is between 0.53 and 0.57. Lower than this threshold range, model specificity decreases faster than model sensitivity increases, which means that the proportion of false positive predictions will increase more rapidly than that of true positive predictions. By contrast, thresholds above this range will see model sensitivity decreasing faster than model specificity, or in other words, the proportion of false negative predictions will increase faster than that of true negative predictions.

However, balanced accuracy, despite being a widely adopted indicator to construct, compare and select best-performing machine learning models, cannot be readily used to assess a model's usefulness or utilities in real-life scenarios. For example, when the probability threshold is set at 0.55, the positive posterior likelihood (LR+) of the selected machine learning classifier (linear SVM with z score normalisation) is 3.58 (95 per cent confidence intervals, C.I. 3.02, 4.23), and its associated posterior probability (odds) are 75 per cent (3.0) (95 per cent C.I. 71 per cent, 78 per cent), based on a prior probability (odds) of 45.2 per cent (0.82) of Japanese translations of low readability in the training dataset used to develop the classifier.

Table 5.6 *Utilities of the best-performing model Linear SVM_7_ZSN under different thresholds*

Thresholds	Sensitivity	Specificity	BA	Positive Likelihood Ratio (LR+)	Positive Posterior Odds *	1 in every x number text with positive result are not readable translations	Negative Likelihood Ratio (LR-)	Negative Posterior Odds	1 in every x number text with negative result are readable translations
0.40	0.89	0.63	0.76	2.36	1.93	1.52	0.18	0.15	1.15
0.41	0.88	0.65	0.76	2.49	2.03	1.49	0.19	0.16	1.16
0.42	0.87	0.67	0.77	2.67	2.18	1.46	0.19	0.16	1.16
0.43	0.86	0.69	0.77	2.75	2.25	1.44	0.21	0.17	1.17
0.44	0.84	0.70	0.77	2.80	2.29	1.44	0.23	0.18	1.18
0.45	0.84	0.71	0.77	2.85	2.33	1.43	0.23	0.19	1.19
0.46	0.84	0.72	0.78	2.95	2.41	1.42	0.23	0.19	1.19
0.47	0.83	0.72	0.77	2.95	2.42	1.41	0.24	0.19	1.19
0.48	0.82	0.72	0.77	2.92	2.39	1.42	0.25	0.20	1.20
0.49	0.80	0.74	0.77	3.05	2.49	1.40	0.27	0.22	1.22
0.50	0.80	0.75	0.77	3.17	2.59	1.39	0.27	0.22	1.22
0.51	0.79	0.75	0.77	3.14	2.57	1.39	0.28	0.23	1.23
0.52	0.79	0.76	0.77	3.26	2.66	1.38	0.28	0.23	1.23
0.53	0.78	0.78	0.78	3.48	2.85	1.35	0.29	0.24	1.24
0.54	0.78	0.79	0.78	3.61	2.95	1.34	0.29	0.23	1.23
0.55	0.77	0.79	0.78	3.58	2.93	1.34	0.29	0.24	1.24
0.56	0.76	0.79	0.78	3.65	2.99	1.34	0.30	0.25	1.25

0.57	0.75	0.80	0.78	3.71	3.03	1.33	0.31	0.25	1.25
0.58	0.74	0.81	0.77	3.85	3.15	1.32	0.32	0.26	1.26
0.59	0.72	0.81	0.76	3.80	3.11	1.32	0.35	0.28	1.28
0.60	0.72	0.82	0.77	3.91	3.20	1.31	0.35	0.29	1.29
0.61	0.71	0.83	0.77	4.10	3.35	1.30	0.36	0.29	1.29
0.62	0.70	0.83	0.77	4.19	3.43	1.29	0.37	0.30	1.30
0.63	0.69	0.84	0.76	4.29	3.51	1.29	0.37	0.31	1.31
0.64	0.68	0.85	0.77	4.56	3.73	1.27	0.38	0.31	1.31
0.65	0.67	0.86	0.77	4.79	3.92	1.26	0.38	0.31	1.31
0.66	0.65	0.87	0.76	4.84	3.96	1.25	0.40	0.33	1.33
0.67	0.65	0.87	0.76	5.02	4.10	1.24	0.41	0.33	1.33
0.68	0.64	0.88	0.76	5.16	4.22	1.24	0.42	0.34	1.34
0.69	0.63	0.89	0.76	5.63	4.61	1.22	0.42	0.34	1.34
0.70	0.62	0.89	0.76	5.68	4.65	1.22	0.43	0.35	1.35
0.71	0.61	0.89	0.75	5.75	4.70	1.21	0.44	0.36	1.36
0.72	0.61	0.90	0.75	6.06	4.96	1.20	0.44	0.36	1.36
0.73	0.60	0.90	0.75	6.18	5.05	1.20	0.44	0.36	1.36
0.74	0.59	0.91	0.75	6.41	5.25	1.19	0.45	0.37	1.37
0.75	0.58	0.91	0.75	6.52	5.33	1.19	0.46	0.38	1.38
0.76	0.55	0.92	0.74	6.68	5.46	1.18	0.49	0.40	1.40
0.77	0.54	0.92	0.73	7.04	5.76	1.17	0.50	0.41	1.41
0.78	0.52	0.92	0.72	6.78	5.55	1.18	0.52	0.42	1.42
0.79	0.52	0.93	0.73	7.52	6.15	1.16	0.52	0.42	1.42
0.80	0.51	0.94	0.73	8.55	6.99	1.14	0.52	0.42	1.42
0.81	0.50	0.95	0.72	9.20	7.53	1.13	0.53	0.44	1.44
0.82	0.48	0.95	0.71	9.25	7.57	1.13	0.55	0.45	1.45
0.83	0.47	0.95	0.71	9.67	7.91	1.13	0.55	0.45	1.45
0.84	0.46	0.95	0.71	10.04	8.22	1.12	0.56	0.46	1.46
0.85	0.45	0.96	0.70	10.37	8.48	1.12	0.58	0.47	1.47

Table 5.6 (*cont.*)

Thresholds	Sensitivity	Specificity	BA	Positive Likelihood Ratio (LR+)	Positive Posterior Odds	1 in every x number text with positive result are not readable translations	Negative Likelihood Ratio (LR-)	Negative Posterior Odds	1 in every x number text with negative result are readable translations
0.86	0.42	0.97	0.69	12.35	10.11	1.10	0.60	0.49	1.49
0.87	0.40	0.97	0.68	13.69	11.20	1.09	0.62	0.51	1.51
0.88	0.38	0.98	0.68	16.44	13.44	1.07	0.64	0.52	1.52
0.89	0.35	0.99	0.67	32.09	26.25	1.04	0.65	0.54	1.54
0.90	0.33	0.99	0.66	30.00	24.54	1.04	0.68	0.55	1.55

*Based on a prior probability (odds) of 45.2 per cent (0.8) from the training dataset.

In practical terms, the posterior probability and the posterior odds of the predictive assessment means that when using this machine learning (ML) classifier (Linear SVM) to predict and detect Japanese translations of disaster information which are below the predefined readability level for the Japanese readers, 100 out of 134 translations which are predicted as positive cases or non-readable translations, will truly lack readability for the target readers (with a readability score equal or lower than 2.5 on the Japanese Text Readability Measurement Scale), whereas thirty-four readable Japanese translations will be mislabelled as non-readable that require further human revision, resulting in extra cost incurred by a relatively small LR+ of 3.58.

As we can see from the table of ML threshold breakdowns, the higher the threshold, the higher the positive predictive likelihood (LR+) and the positive posterior odds, and thus the higher the precision rate of the classifier to detect Japanese translations that are truly below the predefined readability level of 2.5 on the JTRMS scale. The higher the prediction precision rate, the lower the cost of hiring human translators to revise translations. Existing research has recommended positive likelihood ratios (LR+) for model selection, which range between 4 and 10. Again, the selection of an optimal or more importantly, a practically meaningful LR+ depends on the context the machine learning classifiers are developed to improve the cost-effectiveness of human translation revision, and the optimal allocation of limited human translation resources in low-resourced working environments.

In the context of translation quality assessment such as this one on predictive translation readability analyses based on predefined quantitative criteria and insights from applied linguistics and language education, selection of ML models with practically useful positive likelihood ratios (LR+) needs to take into consideration the availability and affordability of human revision. For translation language pairs which are well studied, for which qualified translators are relatively easy to source, LR+ can be shifted towards lower thresholds in the probability breakdown table. However, for minority languages for which qualified translators are scarce, or with very limited funding to support their work, we recommend using LR+ at higher levels to help minimise the cost of human translation revision and post-editing work.

Another important function of predictive translation quality assessment using machine learning classifiers is the prediction of the probability or likelihood ratio of an unassessed translation that is readable for the target readers. This is expressed through the negative posterior odds of a translation, which is contingent upon the prior odds of positive cases, or in this study, Japanese translations of low readability, and the model's negative likelihood ratios (LR-), which captures the ability of ML classifiers to detect negative or risk-free individual texts. As discussed above, LR- is the ratio between false negative cases and true negative cases as predicted by a machine learning classifier. As a result, the lower the LR-, the higher the proportion of truly negative cases among all texts labelled as negative cases by the predictive assessment tool. The table of probability threshold breakdown shows that the lower the probability threshold, the lower the LR-, which means that the higher the percentage of readable translations among all translations labelled as readable ones by the classifier. For example, when setting the model probability threshold at 0.55, the negative likelihood ratio (LR-) is 0.29. Based on a prior odds of 0.45, the posterior odds of the prediction of a negative case is 0.24, which means that among 124 Japanese translations that have been predicted as negative or readable texts, 100 are truly negative cases. When decreasing probability thresholds, model sensitivity increases, and the proportion of false negative cases decreases at a faster rate than that of true negative cases. As a result, negative likelihood ratio (LR-) shrinks, suggesting that an increasingly smaller number of translations will be mislabelled as negative or readable translations when they are not.

The analyses above reveal that choosing probability thresholds has multiple implications in the comparison, selection, and interpretation of machine learning classifiers as highly useful and adaptive predictive tools for translation quality assessment. Model accuracy often peaks within certain ranges of probability thresholds, for example, in the vicinity of 0.5, but model accuracy does not translate to its utilities such as precision detection of positive and negative cases expressed through positive (LR+) and negative likelihood ratios (LR-). Like model sensitivity and specificity pairs, LR+ and LR- exist in pairs and exhibit an inverse relation which has important practical implications for assessing the overall practical usefulness of ML classifiers. Increasing probability thresholds will lead to higher LR+ that are indicative of higher proportions of positive (risk) cases among all positive cases labelled by ML classifiers. Higher positive likelihood ratios can significantly improve the cost-effectiveness of the predictive assessment using automated classifiers. However, increase in probability thresholds can also lead to higher LR- indicating higher proportions of false negative (safe) cases among all negative cases predicted by ML classifiers. Higher negative likelihood ratios will inevitably reduce the reliability of the negative assessment result of ML classifiers, as increasing numbers of complex translations requiring human revision will likely be mislabelled as readable translations for the target audience. Some studies recommend LR- to be lower than 0.2 or even 0.1 to minimise the ratio between false negative and true negative cases.

In the context of predictive translation quality assessment, the selection of a negative likelihood ratio will depend on the nature, or potential harms of positive cases. For example, if the assessment targets clinically significant mistranslations that can cause life-threatening harms to multicultural patients with limited health literacy and English proficiency as the end users of health or medical translations, we recommend more conservative negative likelihood ratios, for example, lower than 0.1 to minimise the rate of false negative predictions. It should be noted that with ML classifiers that have moderate overall accuracy, for example, under 0.9, conservative negative likelihood ratios, which can be attained through lowering probability thresholds, will come at a cost, i.e., the reduced cost-effectiveness of ML classifiers, as the positive likelihood ratio decreases. As explained above, lower positive likelihood ratios will incur additional costs of human revision.

To sum up, the selection of probability thresholds of ML classifiers is a critical step in the proposed predictive translation quality assessment as a decision aid to optimise the design of original English information for translation purposes. A few technical issues need to be taken into consideration when deliberating on the probability threshold for a given ML classifier. With 'perfect' ML classifiers which have an overall balanced accuracy of 0.9 or above, or both sensitivity and specificity draw close to 1.0, it is more likely to identify a shared threshold point at which a very large positive likelihood ratio (larger than 10) and a very small negative likelihood ratio (smaller than 0.1) pair can be both identified. With such ML classifiers, the predictive assessment will be highly reliable and cost-effective, as such ML classifiers will have both very low false negative and false positive rates. However, in real-life scenarios, ML classifiers with moderate performance are more common and practically attainable. Moderate model performance is reflected in its sensitivity and specificity pairs with values ranging between 0.6 to 0.8 under different probability thresholds, as shown in this study. With ML classifiers with moderate sensitivity and specificity pairs, we can adjust probability thresholds to enhance the property and practical function of the classifiers, based on the varying priorities of assessment.

If the main function of the tool is to ascertain whether a certain English text will truly cause complex, non-readable translations, increasing probability thresholds will increase positive likelihood ratios and the posterior odds of a positive case prediction. As a result, a greater proportion of the positive case predictions by ML classifiers will genuinely cause translations of limited readability. However, the interpretation of negative predictions by ML classifiers with higher thresholds requires extra caution, as increased negative likelihood ratios will cause increased posterior odds of negative case predictions, which in turn suggests higher proportions of false negative predictions made by such ML classifiers. By contrast, if the main function of the tool is to ascertain whether an English text can be safely translated into accessible and easy target language, lowering the probability threshold will decrease the model negative likelihood ratios and the posterior odds of a negative case prediction. Since the negative likelihood ratio is the ratio between false negative and true negative cases, small LR- will significantly increase the reliability of the negative case predictions by ML classifiers. Classifiers with lower probability thresholds and smaller positive and negative likelihood ratios can incur higher costs in real-life working environments, when being used for screening English texts unsuitable for producing readable, easy translations in the target language. That is because smaller positive likelihood ratios will lead to higher proportions of false positive cases. Nevertheless, if the English text revision can be conducted in a well-supported, well-funded working environment with adequate staffing of qualified translators, lowering the thresholds to increase the sensitivity of positive predictions and the reliability of negative predictions by ML classifiers can still be justified and practically implemented.

In our study of developing and leveraging predictive tools to optimise the design of English information for multicultural disaster communications, we decided to lower the probability thresholds to reach a negative likelihood ratio around 0.2, as a conservative LR- value. This is based on the following considerations related to the context of the automated predictive translation quality forecasting. First, the nature of positive (risk) cases. Our study focuses on ascertaining the quality and suitability of original English texts for translation and cross-cultural disaster communication purposes. Translations lacking readability can cause misunderstanding of critical disaster information among the Japanese readers. Second, English and Japanese is a well-studied language pair, and qualified translators are relatively easy to source. Despite that lower thresholds and smaller positive likelihood ratios will incur higher costs in engaging professional translators to review, revise English texts labelled as positive cases by ML classifiers, and this is not considered inviable or impractical in real-life scenarios. As a result, we recommend a reference threshold in the vicinity of 0.43 when the negative likelihood ratio (LR-) is controlled at 0.2 or below as a conservative level for ascertaining the suitability of English texts for producing readable disaster translations for Japanese-speaking readers with Year 10 or below education.

The next section demonstrates how to leverage the predictive assessment tools developed to improve the suitability of English texts for translation into readable Japanese, before the actual translation takes place. The predictive assessment process does not assume any prior knowledge of Japanese and can be conducted by domain experts and emergency service providers when designing disaster or environmental health risk information for multicultural readers and can help them develop disaster literacy and self-resilience through readable and comprehensible disaster translations.

5.8 Applying the Predictive Assessment Model to Improve the Translatability of English Disaster Information

A major methodological advantage of machine learning classifiers is that they can help English disaster information developers to predict the probability that the Japanese translation of the English text, before the translation is produced, will be equal or below a predefined acceptable readability level, or in other words, will not be readable for Japanese readers. The predictive assessment is based on the linguistic and textual features of the English text, and takes place before the English text is translated to Japanese. The probabilistic prediction provides an indictive tool to guide and support disaster information developers to iteratively improve the English text and gradually increase its suitability for translation to another language. The suitability of an English text for translation into a readable text in the target language, i.e., Japanese in this study, is expressed through the predicted low posterior probabilities of the undesired binary outcome, which is a translation of low readability that is equal or below the predefined threshold of 2.5 on the JTRMS scale. The technical advantage and convenience of the predictive assessment is that it does not require the English source text to be first translated to Japanese. Disaster information developers can decide whether the English text requires any further revision after the posterior probability has reached a certain level, normally below the selected probability threshold.

Our study set the probability threshold of the machine learning classifier at 0.43, and the predictive assessment tool thus has a positive likelihood (LR+) of 2.75 and a negative likelihood (LR-) of 0.21. If an English text scores a posterior probability higher than 0.43, we will classify the text as a 'risky' case, that is, it is likely to cause a Japanese translation of low readability for a general Japanese-speaking readership. By contrast, if the predictive assessment returns a posterior probability equal or smaller than 0.43, we will treat the English text as a 'safe' case which is unlikely to be translated into a complex, non-readable Japanese text. With English texts of posterior probabilities higher than 0.43, it is recommended that further linguistic and textual revision be conducted. The revision can be based on the features used for the developing machine learning classifiers. Specific textual simplification techniques include reducing English ad-positions (ADP) (O.R.12.537, 95 per cent C.I. 2.001, 78.546, p=0.007), increasing punctuation marks (PUNCT) (O.R. 0.000153, 95 per cent C.I. 0.000033, 0.001, p<.001) and proper nouns (PROPN) (O.R.0.000393, 95 per cent C.I. 0.000098, 0.002, p<.001), and lowering the scores of Danielson-Bryan 1 Grade Level (O.R.3.416, 95 per cent C.I. 2.593, 4.5, p<0.001), Flesch-Kincaid Grade Level (O.R.1.149, 95 per cent C.I. 1.086, 1.217, p<0.001), and Coleman-Liau estimated Cloze scores (O.R. 1.058, 95 per cent C.I. 1.042, 1.074, p<0.001).

Step 1 Initial Predictive Assessment

Table 5.7 shows an original English text with a predicted probability of 0.62, which is above the predefined threshold of 0.43. Recalling that the predicted membership (positive cases) is Japanese translations with readability scores equal or smaller than 2.5, which are classified as non-readable translations. The six linguistic features used to develop the classifier were ADP (ad-positions), PUNCT (punctuations), PROPN (proper nouns), and three readability indexes, i.e., Danielson – Bryan 1 Grade Level, Flesch-Kincaid Grade Level and Coleman-Liau estimated Cloze.

Fagan's nomogram is embedded in the Diagnostic Test Calculator developed by Alan Schwartz of the Department of Medical Education at the University of Illinois at Chicago (http://araw.mede.uic.edu/cgi-bin/testcalc.pl). This calculator is Free Software, available under the Clarified Artistic License. Fagan's nomogram shows the positive posterior probability and the positive posterior odds of the prediction. In Figure 5.4, the left vertical scale shows the prior probability of non-readable Japanese translations, which can be estimated from the dataset collected for developing machine learning classifiers. In our study, the prior probability is 0.452 which means that about half of the English texts are translated into Japanese with readability scores equal or smaller than 2.5. The middle vertical scale exhibits the positive likelihood ratio (LR+) (upper) (4.193) and the negative likelihood ratio (LR-) (lower) (0.365). By linking the prior probability and the positive likelihood ratio (4.193) and extend this line until it intersects with the right vertical scale which indicates the positive

Table 5.7 *Initial predictive assessment of the translatability of the English text*

English Version 1	ADP (Ad-positions)	Punctuation marks (PUNCT)	Proper nouns (PROPN)	Danielson-Bryan 1 Grade Level	Flesch-Kincaid Grade Level	Coleman-Liau estimated Cloze.	Predicted Probability
Crisis Care can help you find crisis accommodation and assist with longer term housing	1	1	1	6.20	9.30	12.70	0.62

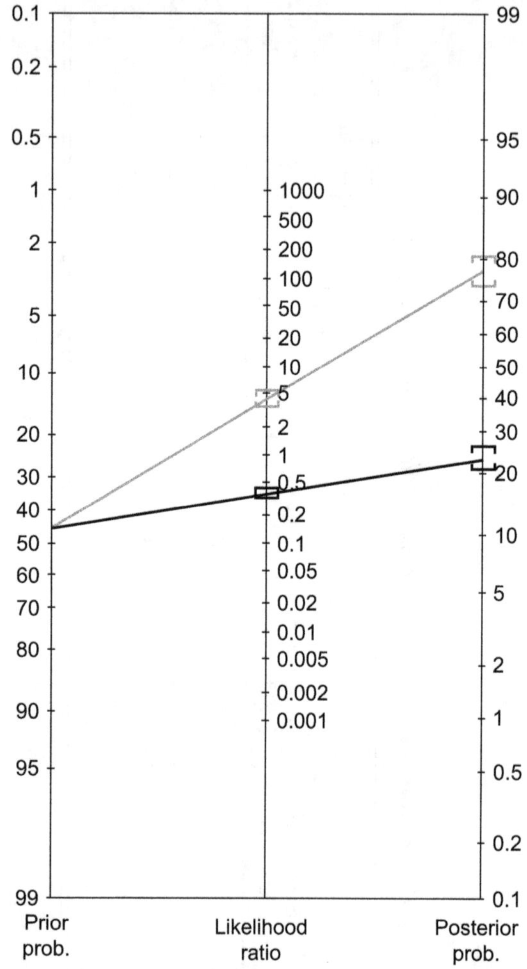

Figure 5.4 Fagan's nomogram (predicted probability=0.62).

posterior probability of the predication. Fagan's nomogram shows that the positive posterior probability is 0.774 and the positive posterior odds is 3.43. This result means that 100 in every 129 English texts with positive results lead to Japanese translations which will have readability scores equal or smaller than 2.5. This result also suggests that about 30 per cent of the positive prediction will be false positive, or English texts which will lead to readable Japanese translations but will be mis-classified as risky cases.

Fagan's nomogram also shows that the negative posterior probability is 0.23 with the negative posterior odds is 0.298. This means that 100 in every 130 English texts with negative results will lead to readable Japanese translation with readability scores larger than 2.5 on the JTRMS scale. Or in other words, about 30 per cent if the negative prediction will be false negative. The trade-off between sensitivity and specificity is an inevitable issue when selecting an optimal probability threshold of a machine learning classifier to increase the practical value of the model.

Step 2 Revision and Reassessment

Table 5.8 shows the linguistic features of the revised English text. By breaking down the original long sentence to two separate sentences, and using shorter, more familiar expressions to replace original more formal expressions, the readability of the English sentence improved significantly. The Danielson-Bryan 1 Grade Level score, Flesch-Kincaid Grade Level and the Coleman-Liau estimated Cloze scores decreased from 6.2, 9.3 and 12.7 to 4.6, 4.2 and 6, respectively. As a result, the predicted probability that the revised English sentence will lead to complex, non-readable Japanese translation also dropped from 0.62 to 0.28. To calculate the posterior probability and odds of the estimation, we again used Fagan's nomogram (Figure 5.5). Since the predicted probability was below the threshold of 0.43, the revised English text was labelled as a negative, 'safe' or translatable sentence. The negative likelihood ratio is 0.103. The prior probability (odds) derived from the training dataset is 45.2 per cent (0.8). By linking the prior probability (45.2) on the left scale and the negative likelihood ratio (0.103) on the middle scale, we arrived at a posterior probability (odds) of 7.8 per cent (0.085) on the right scale on Fagan's nomogram. This result suggests that among every 1000 English texts predicted to be translatable into Japanese or labelled as negative cases, as many as 922 will be truly translated into Japanese with a readability score higher than 2.5 on the JTRMS scale.

Step 3 Verification of the Predictive Assessment Reliability

As a final check of the accuracy and reliability of the machine learning classifier prediction, we produced the Japanese translations by human translators of the two versions of the English text. Table 5.9 shows that as expected, the revised, and simplified English text led to a Japanese translation which had a readability score of 4.82. This was higher than the Japanese readability threshold of 2.5, as well as that of the Japanese translation of the original, more complex English text, which was 2.31.

Table 5.8 *Re-assessment of the suitability of the English text for translation to readable Japanese*

English Version 2	ADP (Ad-positions)	Punctuation marks (PUNCT)	Proper nouns (PROPN)	Danielson-Bryan 1 Grade Level	Flesch-Kincaid Grade Level	Coleman-Liau estimated Cloze.	Predicted Probability
Crisis Care can help you find places to live after crises. They can also find places that you can stay longer.	1	2	1	4.6	4.2	6	0.28

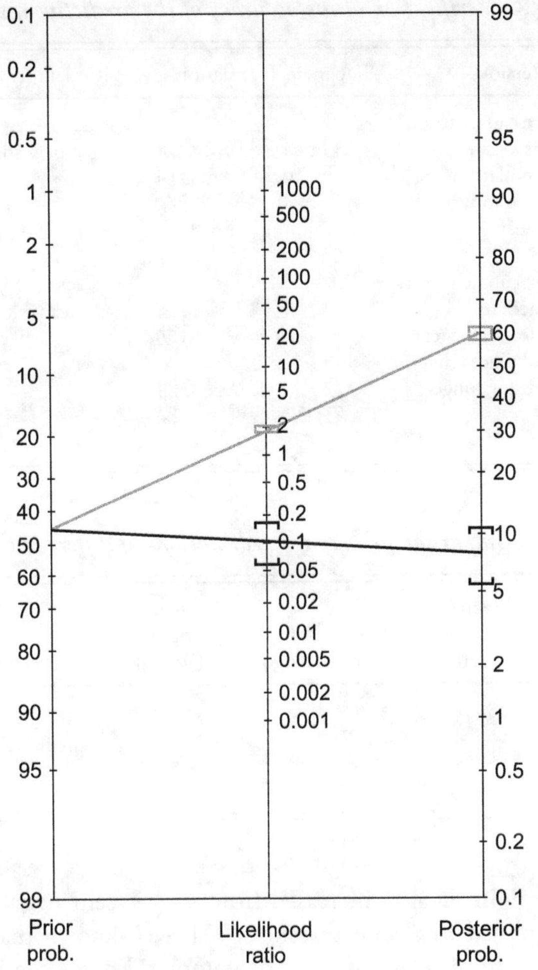

Figure 5.5 Fagan's nomogram (predicted probability=0.28).

On the JTRMS scale, higher scores indicate higher readability of the Japanese texts.

Table 5.10 shows that the revision of the English text had a direct impact on the linguistic profile of the Japanese translations. First, the average sentence length of the Japanese translation decreased by almost a third. Second, the percentage of Japanese words of Chinese origin (Kango) has dropped from 38 per cent to 7 per cent. As a result, the percentage of words

Table 5.9 *Verification of the accuracy of the predictive assessment*

	English Version	Japanese Translation	Readability of Translation
1	Crisis Care can help you find crisis accommodation and assist with longer term housing.	クライシス・ケアは、危機的な状況下での宿泊先を探したり、長期的な住居の斡旋をします	2.31 < 2.5 Not readable translation
2	Crisis Care can help you find places to live after crises. They can also find places that you can stay longer.	クライシス・ケアは、危機の後に住む場所を探す手助けをしてくれる。また、より長く滞在できる場所を探すこともできる。	4.82 > 2.5 Readable translation

Table 5.10 *Comparison of Japanese translations of different English texts*

Japanese translations of	Average sentence length	Chinese-origin words (Kango)	Japanese-origin words (Wago)	Verbs	Auxiliaries
Original English	28	38%	54%	4%	25%
Revised English	16	7%	78%	3%	25%

of Japanese origin (Wago) increased from 54 per cent to 78 per cent to translate simplified English expressions. It is well-known that in written Japanese, the use of Wago instead of complex Kango can significantly improve the readability of the text. Simplifying the original English texts has shifted the use of Wago and Kango in the Japanese translations, as complex, highly formal English terms tend to be translated using Kango in Japanese writing conventions.

5.9 Conclusion

We have demonstrated the application and interpretation of the predictive assessment of the translatability of English disaster information into readable and accessible Japanese. A major methodological advantage of this novel predictive assessment process is that it does not require domain experts developing English disaster information have any prior, in-depth knowledge of the target language of translation. Machine learning classifiers can predict the likelihood that a certain English text will generate a complex Japanese translation, based on the linguistic profile of the English input texts. Using the predictive assessment can significantly improve the cost-effectiveness of developing multicultural and multilingual disaster information which is more readable and accessible for community members or people with limited knowledge of disaster risk reduction and/or general education. It should be noted that when developing and using machine learning classifiers for the purpose of predicting the translatability or suitability of the original English texts for specific readerships from distinct language and cultural backgrounds, classifier accuracy does not translate readability into the practical usefulness of the classifiers. Users of the predictive assessment tools need to select the best probability threshold as the cut-off point for positive and negative predictions in the context of the assessment exercises. Sensitivity and specificity, or positive and negative likelihood ratios exhibit inverse relationships which will have direct impact on the safe and cost-effective use of the automatic assessment tool.

CHAPTER 6

Forecasting Mistakes in Machine Translation of Environmental Health Information to African Languages

6.1 Closing the Gap of Quality of Health Translations to Minority Languages

This chapter introduces a novel translation quality assessment mechanism, which proposes to increase the translatability of English source texts through predictive assessment using machine learning classifiers, before sending the texts for actual translations. The benefits of the pre-editing approach are manifold. First, it will significantly increase the cost-effectiveness of the translation flow, especially for minority languages which often lack adequate staffing of translators and service support in real-life scenarios for migrant communities. Second, translatability enhancement guided by machine learning will help reduce the risks of mistranslations and miscommunications among minorities. Amidst the increasing accessibility of online translation tools and generative artificial intelligence technologies, awareness of the risk of these tools is not enough. Preventative research mechanisms need to be developed to help protect vulnerable communities who are more susceptible to these tools. This chapter offers a practical and viable solution to minimising the risk of mistranslation and misinformation to African minority languages of important environmental health messages. It leverages machine learning and statistics to identify linguistic features of the English health writing which can have a direct impact on the translatability of the English texts to the four African languages under study. The target African languages include Tigrinya, which is an Ethio-Semitic language commonly spoken in Eritrea and in northern Ethiopia's Tigray Region by the Tigrinya and Tigrayan peoples. It is also spoken by the global diaspora of these regions; Somali, is an Afroasiatic language belonging to the Cushitic branch. It is spoken as a mother tongue by Somalis in Greater Somalia and the Somali diaspora. Somali is an official language in Somalia and Ethiopia, and a national language in Djibouti as well as in northeastern Kenya; Swahili, also known by its local name Kiswahili, is a Bantu language spoken by the

Swahili people, who are found primarily in Tanzania, Kenya and Mozambique; and Zulu, which is a Southern Bantu language of the Nguni branch spoken in Southern Africa. It is the language of the Zulu people, with about twelve million native speakers, who primarily inhabit the province of KwaZulu-Natal of South Africa.

6.2 Sources of English Information on Environmental Health

Appendix 6.1 provides the list of texts on health risks from national and international health authorities.

6.3 Linguistic Annotation of the English Source Texts

Tables 6.1 and 6.2 provide the statistics of the corpus created for developing machine learning models.

As detailed in the previous chapter, the same sets of corpus annotation tools were deployed including Readability Studio (Oleander Software) and the semantic annotation system (USAS) developed by Lancaster University.

6.4 Selection of Linguistic Features for Developing Machine Learning Classifiers

Figure 6.1 and Table 6.3 show the result of the logistic regression analysis of the impact of seven linguistic features on the translatability of the English texts to the four African languages under study, i.e., Tigrinya, Zulu, Somali and Swahili. It shows that increasing the use of three linguistic features in the English source texts can significantly reduce the rate of mistranslations into any of the four African languages: percentage of proper nouns (O.R. 0.001, 95 per cent confidence interval, C.I. 0.000, 0.003, $p<0.001$), percentage of

Table 6.1 *Ratios between Part of Speech (POS) categories and the total number of words in the corpus*

ADJ Adjective	ADP Ad-position	ADV Adverb	AUX Auxiliary	CCONJ Coordinating conjunction	NOUN Noun
0.093	0.114	0.029	0.082	0.035	0.276
PART Particle	PRON Pronoun	PROPN Proper Noun	PUNCT Punctuation	SCONJ Subordinating conjunction	VERB Verb
0.026	0.081	0.037	0.134	0.015	0.127

Table 6.2 *Corpus statistics – lexical and textual complexity measures*

Total number of words	Average number of unique words	Average number of characters	Average number of syllables	Average number of numerals	Average number of monosyllabic words
43,170	0.853	4.84	1.589	0.025	0.642
Average number of unique monosyllabic words	Average Number of complex three-syllable words	Average number of unique three-syllable words	Average number of long six-character words	Average number of unique long words	Average frequency in British national corpus (BNC)
0.526	0.149	0.138	0.336	0.305	335.74

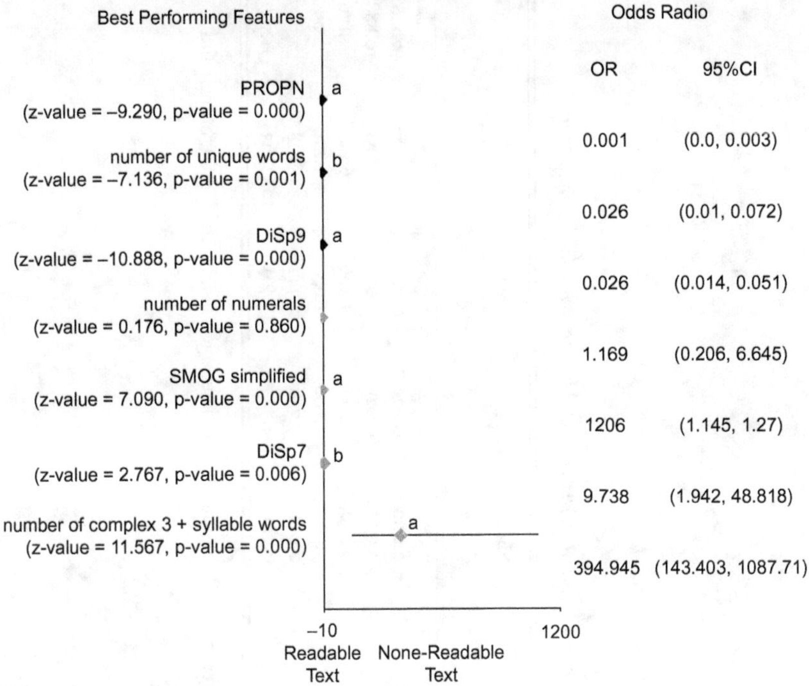

Figure 6.1 Logistic regression forest plot (a: p<0.001, b: p<0.01, c: p<0.05).

unique words (O.R. 0.03, 95 per cent C.I. 0.01, 0.07, p<0.001), and percentage of words in the highest frequent category of words in the BNC spoken corpus, DiSp9 (O.R. 0.03, 95 per cent C.I. 0.01, 0.05, p<0.001). By contrast, the translatability of the English source texts will decrease significantly, when increasing the use of less frequent and more formal words in the BNC spoken corpus, DiSp7 (O.R. 9.74, 95 per cent C.I. 1.94, 48.82, p=0.006), multi-syllable words (O.R. 394.95, 95 per cent C.I. 143.40, 1087.71, p<0.001). Higher scores of the original English texts on the SMOG index also proved a significant predictor of the lack of translatability of the English source text (O.R. 1.21, 95 per cent C.I. 1.15, 1.27, p<0.001).

6.5 Comparing Machine Learning Classifiers

Figure 6.2 and Table 6.4 compare the performance of the machine learning classifiers developed on the testing dataset: support vector

Table 6.3 *Logistic regression analysis of the impact on English features on African translation accuracy*

English Linguistic Features	B	S.E.	Wald	df	Sig.	Exp(B)	95% C. I. for EXP(B)		z-scores
							Lower	Upper	
Per cent of proper nouns	−7.242	0.780	86.304	1	0.000	0.001	0.000	0.003	−9.290
Per cent of unique words	−3.632	0.509	50.811	1	0.000	0.026	0.01	0.072	−7.136
Per cent of DiSp9 words	−3.637	0.334	118.538	1	0.000	0.026	0.014	0.051	−10.888
Per cent of numerals	0.156	0.887	0.031	1	0.860	1.169	0.206	6.645	0.176
SMOG Index score	0.187	0.026	50.264	1	0.000	1.206	1.145	1.270	7.090
Per cent of DiSp7 words	2.276	0.823	7.657	1	0.006	9.738	1.942	48.818	2.767
Per cent of multi-syllable words	5.979	0.517	133.790	1	0.000	394.945	143.403	1087.713	11.567

*The predicted membership is that the English text will cause mistakes in any of the four African languages, i.e., Swahili, Zulu, Somali and Tigrinya.

Table 6.4 *Comparison of machine learning models on the testing data using the DeLong Test*

I	j	AUC difference (i-j)	Variance-corrected t-statistic	Variance-corrected P value*	Probability of i more accurate than j**
LR_ZSN	LR_L2 N	0.031	0.924	0.204	0.796
LR_ZSN	LR_MMN	0.011	0.150	0.444	0.556
LR_ZSN	LR_None	0.016	0.486	0.326	0.674
LR_ZSN	RBF_SVM_L2 N	0.029	0.888	0.212	0.788
LR_ZSN	RBF_SVM_None	0.041	3.013	0.020	0.980

* p values are variance-corrected.
** Bayesian estimation of the comparison result.

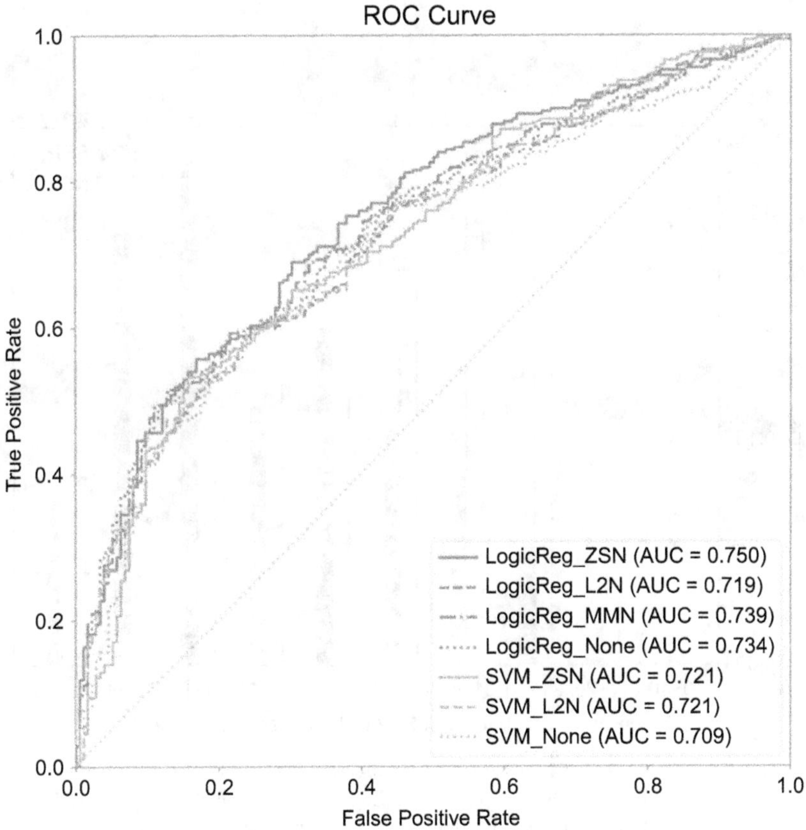

Figure 6.2 Area under the curve of the receiver operating characteristic on the testing dataset.

machine (SVM) with radial basis function kernel (RBF) and logistic regression with seven English linguistic features and three different transformation methods, i.e., z-score (ZSN), min-max normalisation (MMN), and logarithmic normalisation (L2 N). The result shows that regarding the area under the curve of the receiver operating characteristic (ROC), logistic regression with z-score normalisation (LR_ZSN) (AUC=0.750) did not differ significantly from other machine learning classifiers except for RBF_SVM without any data normalisation treatment: LR_L2 N (AUC=0.719, p=0.204), LR_MMN (AUC=0.739, p=0.444), LR_None (AUC=0.734, p=0.212), RBF_SVM_L2 N (AUC=0.721, p=0.212) RBF_SVM_None (AUC=0.709, p=0.020).

Figure 6.3 shows that 61 per cent of English text associated with readable translations were assigned a probability under 51 per cent, and 75 per cent of English text associated with non-readable translations were assigned a probability equal or larger than 50 per cent.

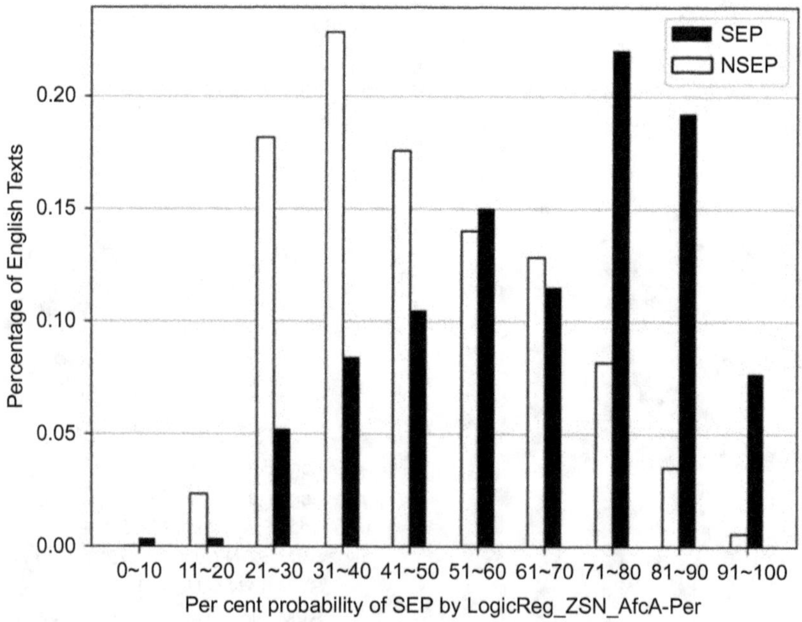

Figure 6.3 Percentage of English texts associated with erroneous and correct African translations assigned by the best performing Logistic Regression classifier with seven linguistic features (LR_7) to each 10 per cent probability bin.

6.6 Setting the Thresholds of Sensitivity and Specificity Pairs of Machine Learning Models

See Table 6.5.

6.7 Predictive Assessment to Improve the Translatability of English Texts to African Languages

Step 1 Initial Predictive Assessment

The first step of the proposed predictive assessment of the translatability of English texts into the African languages under study is to generate the risk probability of an English text excerpt or sentence, that is, how likely the English text will lead erroneous translations in any of the four African languages, if it is subjected to machine translation tools such as Google. The machine learning classifier developed and selected, i.e., logistic regression with seven linguistic features as predicting features, will automatically produce a risk score to aid the decision process. As explained in the section above, to minimise the rate of false negative prediction, that is, an English text which will lead to translation mistakes, but is mislabelled as a 'safe' text for translation use by the classifier, we set the probability threshold at a very low level of 0.21 which has a sensitivity and specificity of 0.993 and 0.029. With such a high sensitivity, the negative likelihood ratio (negative posterior odds) of the selected classifier was controlled at reasonably low level of 0.24 (0.36), which is the lowest level that this classifier can possibly attain. Specifically, this means that if the risk probabilities of 100 English texts are lower than 0.21 or being predicted by the classifier as 'safe' texts for translation use, seventy-five English texts will be truly 'safe' texts, whereas the remaining twenty-five predictions will be false negative cases. Although not perfect, this technique, when applied in the pre-assessment of the translatability of English texts at large scale will prove extremely cost-effective, especially in real-life scenarios when properly trained and qualified health translators proficient in these African minority languages are scare and hard to source.

In this section, we will illustrate the automatic pre-assessment of the risk profile of English environmental health information regarding their translatability into Tigrinya, Zulu, Somali and Swahili languages. The five examples are chosen randomly from the testing database used to test the machine learning classifier. These were written by national and international health authorities and emergency departments. These sentences all had a predicted risk score higher than the threshold of 0.21 and were

Table 6.5 *Utilities of the best-performing model Logistic Regresion_7_ZSN under different thresholds*

Threshold	Sensitivity	Specificity	Positive Likelihood Ratio (LR+)	Positive Posterior Odds*	1 in every x number text with positive result will cause machine translation mistakes	Negative Likelihood Ratio (LR-)	Negative Posterior Odds	1 in every x number text with negative result will not cause machine translation mistakes
0.13	0.993	0.006	1	1.498	1.667	1.17	1.75	2.75
0.14	0.993	0.006	1	1.498	1.667	1.17	1.75	2.75
0.15	0.993	0.006	1	1.498	1.667	1.17	1.75	2.75
0.16	0.993	0.012	1.01	1.508	1.663	0.58	0.875	1.875
0.17	0.993	0.018	1.01	1.517	1.659	0.39	0.583	1.583
0.18	0.993	0.018	1.01	1.517	1.659	0.39	0.583	1.583
0.19	0.993	0.023	1.02	1.525	1.656	0.3	0.457	1.457
0.2	0.993	0.023	1.02	1.525	1.656	0.3	0.457	1.457
0.21	**0.993**	**0.029**	**1.02**	**1.534**	**1.652**	**0.24**	**0.362**	**1.362**
0.22	0.983	0.053	1.04	1.557	1.642	0.32	0.481	1.481
0.23	0.976	0.064	1.04	1.564	1.639	0.38	0.563	1.563
0.24	0.969	0.076	1.05	1.573	1.636	0.41	0.612	1.612
0.25	0.969	0.088	1.06	1.594	1.627	0.35	0.528	1.528
0.26	0.955	0.117	1.08	1.622	1.616	0.38	0.577	1.577
0.27	0.955	0.14	1.11	1.666	1.6	0.32	0.482	1.482
0.28	0.951	0.164	1.14	1.706	1.586	0.3	0.448	1.448
0.29	0.951	0.181	1.16	1.742	1.574	0.27	0.406	1.406
0.3	0.941	0.205	1.18	1.775	1.563	0.29	0.432	1.432
0.31	0.927	0.222	1.19	1.787	1.56	0.33	0.493	1.493
0.32	0.92	0.251	1.23	1.842	1.543	0.32	0.478	1.478

0.33	0.913	0.263	1.24	1.858	1.538	0.33	0.496	1.496
0.34	0.913	0.275	1.26	1.889	1.529	0.32	0.475	1.475
0.35	0.902	0.298	1.28	1.927	1.519	0.33	0.493	1.493
0.36	0.899	0.327	1.34	2.004	1.499	0.31	0.463	1.463
0.37	0.895	0.339	1.35	2.031	1.492	0.31	0.465	1.465
0.38	0.885	0.386	1.44	2.162	1.463	0.3	0.447	1.447
0.39	0.868	0.415	1.48	2.226	1.449	0.32	0.477	1.477
0.4	0.857	0.433	1.51	2.267	1.441	0.33	0.495	1.495
0.41	0.847	0.462	1.57	2.362	1.423	0.33	0.497	1.497
0.42	0.84	0.485	1.63	2.447	1.409	0.33	0.495	1.495
0.43	0.826	0.503	1.66	2.493	1.401	0.35	0.519	1.519
0.44	0.815	0.526	1.72	2.579	1.388	0.35	0.528	1.528
0.45	0.812	0.532	1.74	2.603	1.384	0.35	0.53	1.53
0.46	0.801	0.544	1.76	2.635	1.38	0.37	0.549	1.549
0.47	0.784	0.55	1.74	2.613	1.383	0.39	0.589	1.589
0.48	0.777	0.556	1.75	2.625	1.381	0.4	0.602	1.602
0.49	0.763	0.585	1.84	2.758	1.363	0.41	0.608	1.608
0.5	0.753	0.608	1.92	2.881	1.347	0.41	0.609	1.609
0.51	0.742	0.626	1.98	2.976	1.336	0.41	0.618	1.618
0.52	0.725	0.632	1.97	2.955	1.338	0.44	0.653	1.653
0.53	0.711	0.661	2.1	3.146	1.318	0.44	0.656	1.656
0.54	0.7	0.673	2.14	3.211	1.311	0.45	0.669	1.669
0.55	0.683	0.696	2.25	3.37	1.297	0.46	0.683	1.683
0.56	0.669	0.702	2.24	3.367	1.297	0.47	0.707	1.707
0.57	0.645	0.713	2.25	3.371	1.297	0.5	0.747	1.747
0.58	0.627	0.713	2.18	3.277	1.305	0.52	0.785	1.785
0.59	0.61	0.731	2.27	3.401	1.294	0.53	0.8	1.8
0.6	0.603	0.749	2.4	3.604	1.278	0.53	0.795	1.795
0.61	0.585	0.778	2.64	3.953	1.253	0.53	0.8	1.8

Table 6.5 (*cont.*)

Threshold	Sensitivity	Specificity	Positive Likelihood Ratio (LR+)	Positive Posterior Odds*	1 in every x number text with positive result will cause machine translation mistakes	Negative Likelihood Ratio (LR-)	Negative Posterior Odds	1 in every x number text with negative result will not cause machine translation mistakes
0.62	0.575	0.795	2.8	4.207	1.238	0.53	0.802	1.802
0.63	0.564	0.801	2.83	4.251	1.235	0.54	0.816	1.816
0.64	0.557	0.819	3.08	4.616	1.217	0.54	0.811	1.811
0.65	0.547	0.83	3.22	4.826	1.207	0.55	0.819	1.819
0.66	0.526	0.848	3.46	5.191	1.193	0.56	0.838	1.838
0.67	0.516	0.854	3.53	5.301	1.189	0.57	0.85	1.85
0.68	0.509	0.86	3.64	5.454	1.183	0.57	0.856	1.856
0.69	0.498	0.871	3.86	5.791	1.173	0.58	0.865	1.865
0.7	0.488	0.877	3.97	5.951	1.168	0.58	0.876	1.876
0.71	0.47	0.877	3.82	5.732	1.174	0.6	0.906	1.906
0.72	0.456	0.883	3.9	5.846	1.171	0.62	0.924	1.924
0.73	0.446	0.906	4.74	7.117	1.141	0.61	0.917	1.917
0.74	0.411	0.912	4.67	7.006	1.143	0.65	0.969	1.969
0.75	0.387	0.912	4.4	6.597	1.152	0.67	1.008	2.008
0.76	0.369	0.918	4.5	6.75	1.148	0.69	1.031	2.031
0.77	0.345	0.93	4.93	7.393	1.135	0.7	1.056	2.056
0.78	0.321	0.936	5.02	7.523	1.133	0.73	1.088	2.088
0.79	0.279	0.942	4.81	7.216	1.139	0.77	1.148	2.148
0.8	0.268	0.959	6.54	9.805	1.102	0.76	1.145	2.145
0.81	0.251	0.959	6.12	9.183	1.109	0.78	1.172	2.172

0.82	0.233	0.959	5.68	8.524	1.117	0.8	1.2	2.2
0.83	0.213	0.965	6.09	9.129	1.11	0.82	1.223	2.223
0.84	0.181	0.971	6.24	9.362	1.107	0.84	1.265	2.265
0.85	0.178	0.982	9.89	14.833	1.067	0.84	1.256	2.256
0.86	0.16	0.988	13.33	20	1.05	0.85	1.275	2.275
0.87	0.143	0.988	11.92	17.875	1.056	0.87	1.301	2.301
0.88	0.108	0.994	18	27	1.037	0.9	1.346	2.346
0.89	0.094	0.994	15.67	23.5	1.043	0.91	1.367	2.367
0.9	0.077	0.994	12.83	19.25	1.052	0.93	1.393	2.393
0.91	0.038	0.994	6.33	9.5	1.105	0.97	1.452	2.452

*Based on a prior probability (odds) of 60 per cent (1.5) from the training dataset.

thus identified as risky cases which are likely to cause mistranslations when being translated using online tools. In addition to providing their predicted risk probability score, the machine learning classifier also returned a breakdown of the scores of the seven predicting features which are the percentages of proper nouns (PROPN), unique words, numerals, complex words of three or more syllables, the frequency rank of the word in the spoken component of the British National Corpus (BNC), i.e., DiSp7 and DiSp9, and lastly, the SMOG index score measuring the readability of the English text. These seven features evaluate the complexity of the lexis (percentage of complex words of three or more syllables), information load of the content (percentages of unique words, proper nouns, and numerals), familiarity and formality of the expressions in spoken English (DiSp7 and DiSp9, noting that the higher the rank, the more familiar and more information the English expressions), and the overall readability of the text (the SMOG index). Among them, three features are positively associated with higher translatability of the English text, i.e., the percentages of proper nouns (PROPN) and unique words, and DiSp9; and four features are positively associated with lower translatability of the English text, which are the percentages of unique words, complex words of three or more syllables, less familiar, formal expressions within the seventh rank of the BNC spoken corpus component (DiSp7) and the SMOG index. Through providing a detailed breakdown of the linguistic profile of the text (Tables 6.6 to 6.1), English writers of developing information for community translation purposes can concentrate their revision efforts in areas which can effectively improve the translatability of the English text. For example, by means of increasing the percentage of words and expressions which are positively associated with higher English text translatability, or reducing the use of expressions which are contributors to the lack of translatability of English texts. Examples 6.1 to 6.5 are taken from the website of the WHO.

Example 6.1 (0.24) (See Table 6.6)

The growth of the bacteria and the formation of toxin occur in products with low oxygen content and certain combinations of storage temperature and preservative parameters. This happens most often in lightly preserved foods and in inadequately processed, home-canned or home-bottled foods.

Source of information: https://www.who.int/news-room/fact-sheets/detail/botulism

Table 6.6 *Linguistic profile statistics – Example 6.1*

Total words	44
Per cent of proper nouns	0.0
Per cent of unique words	0.75
Per cent of DiSp9 words	0.318
Per cent of numerals	0.0
SMOG Index score	14
Per cent of DiSp7 words	0.0909
Per cent of multi-syllable words	0.182
Predicted probability of potentially causing machine translation (MT) mistakes	0.24

Example 6.2 (0.237) (See Table 6.7)

If exposure to the toxin via aerosol inhalation is suspected, additional exposure to the patient and others must be prevented. The patient's clothing must be removed and stored in plastic bags until it can be washed thoroughly with soap and water. The patient should shower and be decontaminated immediately.

Source of information: https://www.who.int/news-room/fact-sheets/detail/botulism

Table 6.7 *Linguistic profile statistics – Example 6.2*

Total words	50
Per cent of proper nouns	0.0
Per cent of unique words	0.7
Per cent of DiSp9 words	0.44
Per cent of numerals	0.0
SMOG Index score	13
Per cent of DiSp7 words	0.06
Per cent of multi-syllable words	0.2
Predicted probability of potentially causing MT mistakes	0.237

Example 6.3 (0.24) (See Table 6.8)

During land inundation tsunami inundation is widespread and extends to areas not normally submerged by water. Tsunami waves can run up well beyond the high tide mark, in extreme cases up to a kilometre inland or up to 10 metres above sea level. Tsunami can also extend into harbours, rivers and estuaries. This is why tsunami safety advice for a tsunami with land inundation threat states that you should move away from low lying coastal areas, harbours and estuaries as soon as a Tsunami Warning is issued.

Source: www.ses.nsw.gov.au/tsunami-resources/before-a-tsunami/know-your-risk/

Table 6.8 *Linguistic profile statistics – Example 6.3*

Total words	86
Per cent of proper nouns	0.058
Per cent of unique words	0.733
Per cent of DiSp9 words	0.302
Per cent of numerals	0.012
SMOG Index score	13
Per cent of DiSp7 words	0.058
Per cent of multi-syllable words	0.163
Predicted probability of potentially causing MT mistakes	0.24

Example 6.4 (0.375) (See Table 6.9)

Prevention or reduction of human exposure is best done via source-directed measures, i.e., strict control of industrial processes to reduce formation of dioxins as much as possible. This is the responsibility of national governments.

Source of information: https://www.who.int/news-room/fact-sheets/detail/dioxins-and-their-effects-on-human-health

Table 6.9 *Linguistic profile statistics – Example 6.4*

Total words	37
Per cent of proper nouns	0.0
Per cent of unique words	0.865
Per cent of DiSp9 words	0.216
Per cent of numerals	0.0
SMOG Index score	16
Per cent of DiSp7 words	0.108
Per cent of multi-syllable words	0.324
Predicted probability of potentially causing MT mistakes	0.375

Example 6.5 (0.381) (See Table 6.10)

Unnecessary transfusions and unsafe transfusion practices expose patients to the risk of serious adverse transfusion reactions and transfusion-transmissible infections. Unnecessary transfusions also reduce the availability of blood products for patients who are in need.

Source: https://www.who.int/news-room/fact-sheets/detail/blood-safety-and-availability

Table 6.10 *Linguistic profile statistics – Example 6.5*

Total words	35
Per cent of proper nouns	0.0
Per cent of unique words	0.771
Per cent of DiSp9 words	0.286
Per cent of numerals	0.0
SMOG Index score	16
Per cent of DiSp7 words	0.086
Per cent of multi-syllable words	0.343
Predicted probability of potentially causing MT mistakes	0.381

Step 2 Revision and Reassessment

The second step of the predictive assessment and editing is to revise the original English text to bring its risk probability score lower than the threshold of 0.21. The seven predictive features are indicative of the level of translatability of the English text and its revisions. In this section, we illustrate the revision process and the specific revision strategies used.

Table 6.11 shows the differences between the original sentence of Example 6.1 and its revision. After revision, the risk probability of the text decreased from 0.24 to 0.175, which was below the threshold of 0.21. Table 6.12 shows that the revised text had a higher percentage of unique words (0.914) compared to that of the original sentence (0.75), and the percentage of familiar, informal expressions in spoken English (DiSp9) increased from 0.318 to 0.514. For example, the revision introduced words and word clusters in the category of DiSp9, such as 'can grow', 'kept at', 'at home'. These two features, i.e., unique words and DiSp9 are positively associated with the translatability of English texts. At the same time, the revised text reduced scores of features which are negatively associated with the translatability of English texts. The SMOG index score decreased from Year 14 to Year 9 as the minimal level of education to comprehend the text, and the percentage of complex words containing three or more syllables dropped from 0.182 to 0.086. This includes multi-syllable words such as formation, combinations, preservative, parameters, inadequately, which were either replaced or removed in the revision, without altering or omitting the key messages in the original text. The revised text also had a lower percentage (0.029) of less familiar and more formal expressions in the word list of DiSp7, compared to that of the original text (0.0909). Translatability enhancement is not limited to

Table 6.11 *Linguistic profile statistics – Revised text of Example 6.1*

	Revision	Original
	Bacteria and other toxic content can grow in food kept at some temperatures or using certain ways to store them. This will not happen when food is stored properly with cans or bottles at home.	The growth of the bacteria and the formation of toxin occur in products with low oxygen content and certain combinations of storage temperature and preservative parameters. This happens most often in lightly preserved foods and in inadequately processed, home-canned or home-bottled foods.
Total words	35	44
Per cent of proper nouns	0	0
Per cent of unique words	0.914	0.75
Per cent of DiSp9 words	0.514	0.318
Per cent of numerals	0	0
SMOG Index score	9	14
Per cent of DiSp7 words	0.029	0.0909
Per cent of multi-syllable words	0.086	0.182
Predicted probability of potentially causing MT mistakes	0.175	0.24

the lexical level. Highly complex structures of the original text were rephrased and simplified. For example, 'products with certain combinations of storage temperature and preservative parameters' was rephrased as 'food kept at some temperatures or using certain ways to store them', or 'this happens most often in lightly preserved foods and in inadequately processed' was rephrased as 'This will not happen when food is stored properly'.

Table 6.13 shows another revision strategy which focuses on reducing the use of complex and less familiar expressions in spoken English. First, decrease the percentage of complex words containing three or more syllables from 0.2 to 0.02, such as exposure, inhalation, suspected, additional, prevented, thoroughly, decontaminated, and immediately. Second, decrease the percentage of formal, less familiar expressions in the category of DiSp7 from 0.06 to 0.028. Third, increase the readability

Table 6.12 *Linguistic profile statistics – Revised text of Example 6.2*

	Revision	Original
	When someone has breathed in toxic aerosol, they should avoid more contact with the toxin. Their clothing must be put in a plastic bag, washed with soap and water. They also need to bathe, clean well.	If exposure to the toxin via aerosol inhalation is suspected, additional exposure to the patient and others must be prevented. The patient's clothing must be removed and stored in plastic bags until it can be washed thoroughly with soap and water. The patient should shower and be decontaminated immediately.
Total words	36	50
Per cent of proper nouns	0	0
Per cent of unique words	0.917	0.7
Per cent of DiSp9 words	0.444	0.44
Per cent of numerals	0	0
SMOG Index score	6	13
Per cent of DiSp7 words	0.028	0.06
Per cent of multi-syllable words	0.02	0.2
Predicted probability of potentially causing MT mistakes	0.204	0.237

of the English text, as the minimal education level required to read the text decreased from Year 13 to Year 6. As a result, the predicted probability of the original English text causing mistranslations reduced from 0.237 to 0.204, which was slightly below the predefined threshold of 0.21. Highly complex structures of the original text were rephrased and simplified. For example, 'if exposure to the toxin via aerosol inhalation is suspected' was rephrased as 'when someone has breathed in toxic aerosol', or 'additional exposure to the patient and others must be prevented' was changed for a non-passive phrase 'they (patients) should avoid more contact with the toxin', or 'the patient should shower and be decontaminated immediately' was revised for a more actional and direct advice 'they also need to bathe, clean well'.

Table 6.13 *Linguistic profile statistics – Revised text of Example 6.3*

	Revision	Original
	Tsunami can cause flood on the land. Its waves can reach areas that are normally dry and get much higher than normal tides. The water can run a kilometre into the land, or ten metres above the sea level. Tsunami also gets to harbours, rivers. When you hear that an upcoming tsunami may come ashore, you must leave those risky places quickly.	During land inundation tsunami inundation is widespread and extends to areas not normally submerged by water. Tsunami waves can run up well beyond the high tide mark, in extreme cases up to a kilometre inland or up to 10 metres above sea level. Tsunami can also extend into harbours, rivers, and estuaries. This is why tsunami safety advice for a tsunami with land inundation threat states that you should move away from low lying coastal areas, harbours, and estuaries as soon as a Tsunami Warning is issued.
Total words	62	86
Per cent of proper nouns	0.032	0.058
Per cent of unique words	0.839	0.733
Per cent of DiSp9 words	0.355	0.302
Per cent of numerals	0	0.012
SMOG Index score	9	13
Per cent of DiSp7 words	0.048	0.058
Per cent of multi-syllable words	0.097	0.163
Predicted probability of potentially causing MT mistakes	0.201	0.24

Table 6.13 provides another illustration of the pre-editing and revision process, which is guided and supported by the machine learning prediction technique. The revised text has fewer proper nouns such as tsunami, but the shorter total length of the sentence increased the content richness as indicated by the percentage of unique words from 0.733 to 0.839. The revision also introduced more familiar expressions as highly frequent

words in the BNC spoken corpus, DiSp9, which increased from 0.302 to 0.355. The percentage of complex, multi-syllable words decreased from 0.163 to 0.097 by replacing formal words such as 'inundation', 'submerged' with 'flood', 'dry', and removing adjectives without altering or omitting the key messages of the original text such as 'widespread', 'low lying', 'in extreme cases'. Another revision strategy introduced is to paraphrase words or expressions which may lack linguistic and cultural equivalence in the target African languages, such as 'high tide mark', 'inland', 'estuaries', 'tsunami safety advice'. These technical expressions are familiar for English-speaking people, especially those with advanced tsunami and natural disaster prevention mechanisms and infrastructures, but their translations to African minority languages can significantly heighten the risk of mistranslations and miscommunications. To explain and deliver the key messages of the original text without these technical jargons, the revised text restructured and simplified the original text. For example, 'inland tsunami inundation' was explained as 'tsunami can cause flood on the land'. To explain the term 'high tide mark', the revision described it as 'tsunami waves can get much higher than normal tides'. The term 'estuary' was removed from the revision, as it lacks a functional, cultural equivalent in the four African languages under study. The highly complex structure of the original text 'tsunami safety advice for a tsunami with land inundation threat' was replaced with a less formal but more actionable and understandable phrase 'when you hear that an upcoming tsunami may come ashore.'

Table 6.14 shows an example of revising English texts that contain complex multi-syllable expressions, abstract concepts and names of chemicals which lack established translation equivalents in the target African languages. When pre-editing English texts exhibiting such complex linguistic profiles with a predicted probability of causing machine translation mistake of 0.375, higher than the threshold of 0.21, the revision introduced more familiar expressions in the BNC spoken corpus – the percentage of DiSp9 increased from 0.216 to 0.487, and a decrease in formal, less frequent words in the BNC spoken corpus – the percentage of DiSp7 decreased from 0.108 to 0.054. The shift towards using more familiar expressions, as measured by these two indicators, DiSp7and DiSp9, also underlines the rewriting strategy devised in the revision to increase the translatability of the original text to African languages. For example, contrary to the highly formal style of the original text, the revision adopted a more narrative style which naturally introduced more words in the DiSp9 category such as 'can be done through', or 'that are hard to break down

Table 6.14 *Linguistic profile statistics – Revised text of Example 6.4*

	Revision	Original
	Human exposure to environmental pollutants may be avoided or reduced. This can be done through preventing the formation of environmental pollutants that are hard to break down during the industrial process. National governments are responsible for this.	Prevention or reduction of human exposure is best done via source-directed measures, i.e., strict control of industrial processes to reduce formation of dioxins as much as possible. This is the responsibility of national governments.
Total words	37	37
Per cent of proper nouns	0	0
Per cent of unique words	0.811	0.865
Per cent of DiSp9 words	0.487	0.216
Per cent of numerals	0	0
SMOG Index score	13	16
Per cent of DiSp7 words	0.054	0.108
Per cent of multi-syllable words	0.324	0.324
Predicted probability of potentially causing MT mistakes	0.149	0.375

during the'. These two simplified sentence structures were used to redesign the complex original sentence structures that are prone to machine translation mistakes, i.e., 'best done via source-directed measures, i.e., strict control of industrial processes to . . . ', and to replace the original pollutant name 'dioxins' with a clear and concise definition, 'environmental pollutants that are hard to break down' to minimise the risk of miscommunication when the translation of the term 'dioxins' do not a consistent, well established translation equivalents in the African target languages of Tigrinya and Swahili.

The revision also broke the long sentence into two shorter sentences, which helped to bring down the SMOG score from Year 16 to Year 13, despite that the percentage of complex, multi-syllable words remained at the same level of 0.324. Translatability enhancement was also achieved through paraphrasing English expressions lacking suitable and adequate linguistic equivalents in the target African languages due to distinct social and cultural contexts. For example, 'source-directed measures' was removed, as its removal did not affect the delivery of the key message. The name of the chemical 'dioxin' does not have an established scientific translation in Tigrinya and Swahili and was often mistranslated as dioxide. Therefore, the revision provided a more accessible, safe definition of dioxin to remove this translation barrier 'environmental pollutants that are hard to break down' into African minority languages.

Table 6.15 illustrates the revision strategies developed to overcome language barriers in health translation. Specifically, the translation challenge stems from the writing style of the original sentence that is loaded with technical jargons, some of which lack consistent, established equivalents in the target African languages, for example, the key word 'transfusions' lacks accurate translations in two of the four African languages under study and were translated as 'infusions' in Somali and 'blood

Table 6.15 *Linguistic profile statistics – Revised text of Example 6.5*

	Unneeded and unsafe blood transfers are harmful. They can lead to severe reactions or infections caused by blood transfer. Patients in need may thus have less access to blood supply.	Unnecessary transfusions and unsafe transfusion practices expose patients to the risk of serious adverse transfusion reactions and transfusion-transmissible infections. Unnecessary transfusions also reduce the availability of blood products for patients who are in need.
Total words	30	35
Per cent of proper nouns	0	0
Per cent of unique words	0.9	0.771
Per cent of DiSp9 words	0.3	0.286
Per cent of numerals	0	0
SMOG Index score	8	16
Per cent of DiSp7 words	0.067	0.086
Per cent of multi-syllable words	0.1	0.343
Predicted probability of potentially causing MT mistakes	0.203	0.381

clotting' or 'arterial practices' in Swahili. The breakdown of the linguistic profile of the original text shows that two main risk factors which were closely related, i.e., the high SMOG Index score (Year 16), and the high proportion of complex, multi-syllable words (0.343). The revision thus focused on paraphrasing the original text with minimal technical jargons and a simpler, less formal narrative style. The word 'transfusions' was replaced with 'blood transfer', and 'transfusion-transmissible infections' were described as 'infections caused by blood transfer', and 'reduce the availability of blood products' was rephrased as 'have less access to blood supply'. As a result, the percentage of formal expressions in the category of DiSp7 decreased from 0.086 to 0.067, and the percentage of multi-syllable words reduced by 70 per cent from 0.343 to 0.1. Other indicators however remained comparable to those of the original text. The predicted probability of the revision causing mistranslation in any of the four African languages thus dropped from 0.381 to 0.203, which was below the predefined cut-off point of 0.21.

Step 3 Verification of the Predicted Susceptibility to Translation Errors of English Texts

In this section, we will verify the level of translatability of the revised sentences compared to the original ones. Specifically, the comparison will ascertain whether the revision guided by the predictive assessment has reduced the rate of mistranslations to the target African languages by machine translation tools. As explained above, the probability threshold was set at 0.21 to minimise the rate of false negative predictions after the revision of the original text to improve its translatability into any of the four African languages under study. English texts with predicted probability equal or smaller than 0.21 were labelled as 'safe' texts which were unlikely to cause mistakes when translated into any of the four African languages using online translation tools like Google. By contrast, if English texts with predicted probability larger than 0.21 were labelled as 'risky' texts which required further revision to reduce their likelihood of being mistranslated using automatic online tools. Forward translations were produced using Google Translate, and backward translations were produced using Microsoft Bing Translation to verify the consistency, accuracy and reliability of machine translations produced by Google. The use of these online translation tools was between April and August 2023. Tables 6.16 to 6.20 compared original English texts which had caused mistranslations with revised English texts leading to more accurate translations.

Table 6.16 *Verification of predicted susceptibility to translation errors of Example 6.1 and revision*

Predicted probability of causing mistakes in any of the four African languages	**Original English Text** Predicted Risk Probability: 0.24 The growth of the bacteria and the formation of toxin occur in products with low oxygen content and certain combinations of storage temperature and preservative parameters. This happens most often in lightly preserved foods and in inadequately processed, home-canned or home-bottled foods.	**Revised English Text** Predicted Risk Probability: 0.175 Bacteria and other toxic content can grow in food kept at some temperatures or using certain ways to store them. This will not happen when food is stored properly with cans or bottles at home.
Back translation of Tigrinya translation	The growth of the bacteria and the creation of poisons occur in low oxygen concentrations and a combination of products with storage heat and storage standards, which often occur in light-stored foods and in unsuspidated processes, in cans or packaged at home in glass.	Bacteria and other toxic content can be grown in foods stored at certain temperatures or in certain ways, not when food is stored at home with a can or glass.
Back translation of Somali translation	Bacterial growth and toxin formation occur in products with lower oxygen and a combination of storage temperature and protection parameters. This often happens with spicy preserved and inadequately processed, canned foods or home-mixed foods.	Bacteria and other toxic products can grow in food held at some temperature or using specific methods of storage. This does not happen when food is properly stored in cans or bottles at home.
Back translation of Swahili translation	Bacterial growth and toxic formulation occur in products with low oxygen content and	Bacteria and other toxic content can grow in food kept at a certain temperature or use

Table 6.16 (*cont.*)

	a certain combination of storage temperature and storage parameters. This happens most often in less frozen foods and in unwholesome, homemade or bottled homemade foods.	certain methods to store them. This will not happen when food is stored properly with cans or bottles at home.
Back translation of Zulu translation	Bacterial growth and toxic composition occur in low-oxygen products as well as certain combinations of final temperature and storage parameters. This often occurs in low-preserved foods and insufficiently digested foods, which are placed in a home or household bottle.	Bacteria and other toxic content can grow in foods stored at certain temperatures or using certain storage methods. This will not happen if food is stored properly with cans or bottles at home.

Table 6.17 *Verification of predicted susceptibility to translation errors of Example 6.2 and revision*

Predicted probability of causing mistakes in any of the four African languages	**Original English Text** Predicted Risk Probability: 0.237	**Revised English Text** Predicted Risk Probability: 0.204
	If exposure to the toxin via aerosol inhalation is suspected, additional exposure to the patient and others must be prevented. The patient's clothing must be removed and stored in plastic bags until it can be washed thoroughly with soap and water. The patient should shower and be decontaminated immediately.	When someone has breathed in toxic aerosol, they should avoid more contact with the toxin. Their clothing must be put in a plastic bag, washed with soap and water. They also need to bathe, clean well.
Back translation of Tigrinya translation	If exposure to the toxin via respiratory aerosol is suspected, further exposure should protect the patient and others.	Once a person has breathed toxic aerosols, they should avoid contact with the poison, their cloths should be placed

Table 6.17 (*cont.*)

	The patient's clothes should be removed and stored in plastic bags as long as they can be washed with good water and soap. The patient should take a shower and be removed immediately.	in a plastic bag, they should be washed with water and soap, they need to wash, they need to clean well.
Back translation of Somali translation	If toxic exposure to aerosol inhalation is suspected, further exposure to the patient and others should be prevented. The patient's clothes should be removed and stored in a bag so long as they are thoroughly washed with soap and water. The patient should bathe and get dirty immediately.	When someone inhales a toxic aerosol, they should avoid further contact with the toxin. Their clothes should be put in a bag, washed with soap and water. They also need to wash, clean properly.
Back translation of Swahili translation	If it is suspected to be exposure to the toxin through inhalation of aerosol fumes, additional exposure to the patient and others must be prevented. The patient's clothes must be removed and stored in plastic bags until they can be properly washed with soap and water. The patient should be showered and cleaned immediately.	When a person has breathed a toxic aerosol, they should avoid further contact with the toxins. Their clothes must be put in a plastic bag, washed with soap and water. They also need to shower, clean properly.
Back translation of Zulu translation	If it is suspected that exposure is toxic by aerosol exposure, further exposure to the patient and so on should be avoided. The patient's clothes should be removed and stored in plastic bags and thoroughly washed with soap and water. The patient should wash and disinfect immediately.	If a person inhales a toxic aerosol, they should avoid contact with this substance. Their clothes should be placed in a plastic bag, soaked with soap and water. They also need to wash, clean well.

Table 6.18 *Verification of predicted susceptibility to translation errors of Example 6.3 and revision*

Predicted probability of causing mistakes in any of the 4 African language	**Original English Text** Predicted Risk Probability: 0.240	**Revised English Text** Predicted Risk Probability: 0.201
	During land inundation, tsunami inundation is widespread and extends to areas not normally submerged by water. Tsunami waves can run up well beyond the high tide mark, in extreme cases up to a kilometre inland or up to 10 metres above sea level. Tsunami can also extend into harbours, rivers and estuaries. This is why tsunami safety advice for a tsunami with land inundation threat states that you should move away from low lying coastal areas, harbours and estuaries as soon as a Tsunami Warning is issued.	Tsunami can cause flood on the land. Its waves can reach areas that are normally dry and get much higher than normal tides. The water can run a kilometre into the land, or ten metres above the sea level. Tsunami also gets to harbours, rivers. When you hear that an upcoming tsunami may come ashore, you must leave those risky places quickly.
Back translation of Tigrinya translation	During a landslide, tsunamis spread widely and spread to normal, flood-free areas. Tsunami waves can run far beyond the sign of flooding, in extreme conditions up to a mile inland or as high as 10 feet above sea level. Tsunamis can also spread to ports, rivers and floods, which is why tsunami safety advice for land-threatening tsunamis is that you should stay away from low coastal areas, ports and floods as soon as possible.	Tsunamis can cause flooding on the land, its waves can reach normal dry areas and become much higher than normal floods. The water could run a mile to the ground or ten feet above sea level. Tsunamis reach ports, rivers, and you'll have to evacuate the danger areas as soon as you hear that incoming tsunamis could come to the shore.

Table 6.18 (*cont.*)

Back translation of Somali translation	During ground flow, the tsunami flow is pervasive and reaches areas where water does not normally drop. Tsunami waves can be considerably farther away from the oceanic mark, in severe conditions up to one kilometre inland or up to 10 meters above sea level. The tsunami can also spread to ports, rivers and surroundings. This is why tsunami safety advice for tsunamis with land flood risks you should move out of low-lying areas of the coast, ports and surrounding areas as soon as a Tsunami Warning is issued.	A tsunami can cause flooding on the ground. Its waves can reach normally withered areas far above normal waves. The water can run one kilometre on land, or ten metres above sea level. Tsunami also reaches ports, rivers. Once you hear that an upcoming tsunami can come to shore, you should soon abandon those dangerous areas.
Back translation of Swahili translation	During landslides, tsunami flooding spreads and spreads to areas that are not normally submerged by water. Tsunami waves can go as high as the high tide mark, in extreme cases up to one kilometre inland or up to 10 meters above sea level. Tsunamis can also spread across ports, rivers and rivers. That's why the tsunami safety advisory for tsunamis with a threat of land flooding says that you should evacuate from coastal plains, ports and water gates as soon as a Tsunami Warning is issued.	Tsunamis can cause flooding on land. Its waves can reach areas that are normally dry and get higher than normal waves. Water can run one kilometre on land, or ten meters above sea level. Tsunamis also reach ports, rivers. When you hear that an oncoming tsunami could come ashore, you have to leave that dangerous place quickly.
Back translation of Zulu translation	During landslides, tsunami flooding spreads and spreads to rare areas to be	A tsunami could cause flooding on the ground. Its waves can reach areas

Table 6.18 (*cont.*)

	submerged. Tsunami waves can run past the signal of high waves, in extreme conditions up to a mile in the middle of the country or 10 meters above sea level. A tsunami can pass through ports, rivers and river areas. This is why the tsunami safety advice for a tsunami at risk of landslides says it should move away from low-lying coastal areas, ports and port areas immediately after the tsunami warning is issued.	that are usually dry and much higher than normal waves. Water can run a mile on land, or ten meters above sea level. The tsunami has also reached ports, rivers. When you hear that an impending tsunami might come ashore, you should leave those dangerous places immediately.

Table 6.19 *Verification of predicted susceptibility to translation errors of Example 6.4 and revision*

Predicted probability of causing mistakes in any of the four African languages	**Original English Text** Predicted Risk Probability: 0.375	**Revised English Text** Predicted Risk Probability: 0.149
	Prevention or reduction of human exposure is best done via source-directed measures, i.e., strict control of industrial processes to reduce formation of dioxins as much as possible. This is the responsibility of national governments.	Human exposure to environmental pollutants may be avoided or reduced. This can be done through preventing the formation of environmental pollutants that are hard to break down during the industrial process. National governments are responsible for this.
Back translation of Tigrinya translation	Prevention or reduction of human exposure is the best separately-directed measures – strict regulation of industrial processes to reduce the	Human exposure to environmental pollutants can be avoided or reduced, which can be done by preventing environmental

Table 6.19 (*cont.*)

	creation of dioxide as much as possible– the responsibility of national governments.	pollutants that are difficult to break down in the industrial process, and national governments are responsible for this.
Back translation of Somali translation	Preventing or reducing exposure to humans is best done by using eye-guided tiles, for example, strict control of industrial processes to reduce the formation of dioxins as far as possible. This is the responsibility of national governments.	Human exposure to environmental pollution may be avoided or reduced. This can be done by preventing the formation of environmental pollutants that are difficult to break down during the industrial process. National governments are responsible for this.
Back translation of Swahili translation	Preventing or limiting human exposure is best done through source-oriented measures, i.e., strict regulation of industrial processes to limit the formation of as much dioxide as possible. This is the responsibility of the national governments.	Human exposure to pollution can be avoided or minimised. This can be done by preventing the creation of pollution that is difficult to break down during the manufacturing process. National governments are responsible for this.
Back translation of Zulu translation	Preventing or reducing a person's exposure is best done with steps directed at the source, that is, strict control of industrial processes to reduce the formation of dioxins as much as possible. This is the work of national government.	Human exposure to pollutants may be avoided or reduced. This can be done by preventing the formation of pollutants that are difficult to break down during the industrial process. National governments are responsible for this.

Table 6.20 *Verification of predicted susceptibility to translation errors of Example 6.5 and revision*

Predicted probability of causing mistakes in any of the four African languages	**Original English Text** Predicted Risk Probability: 0.381	**Revised English Text** Predicted Risk Probability: 0.203
	Unnecessary transfusions and unsafe transfusion practices expose patients to the risk of serious adverse transfusion reactions and transfusion-transmissible infections. Unnecessary transfusions also reduce the availability of blood products for patients who are in need.	Unneeded and unsafe blood transfers are harmful. They can lead to severe reactions or infections caused by blood transfer. Patients in need may thus have less access to blood supply.
Back translation of Tigrinya translation	Unnecessary blood transfusions and unsafe blood transfusions expose patients to the risk of severe adverse blood transfusions and blood-borne infections, and unnecessary blood transfusions reduce access to blood education for needy patients.	Unnecessary and unsafe blood transfusions are harmful; they can cause serious reactions or infections caused by blood transfusions, thus reducing the chance of patients receiving blood supplies.
Back translation of Somali translation	Unnecessary infusions and practices of non-safe infusion expose the patient to the risk of serious transfusion reactions and infected infected with infusion. Unnecessary infusions also reduce access to blood products for patients in need.	Unnecessary and non-safe blood transfusions are harmful. They can lead to severe reactions or infections caused by blood transfer. Patients who need it may therefore have less chance of getting the blood.
Back translation of Swahili translation	Unnecessary blood clotting and unsafe arterial practices expose patients to the risk of adverse arterial reactions and potential infections. Unnecessary vascularisation also	Unnecessary and unsafe blood transfusion is dangerous. They can cause severe reactions or infections caused by blood transfer. Patients in need may have limited

Table 6.20 (*cont.*)

	reduces access to blood products for patients in need.	access to the blood supply.
Back translation of Zulu translation	Unnecessary blood transfusions and unsafe transfusion procedures put patients at risk of severe reactions and infection of communicable diseases. Unnecessarily injecting blood reduces the availability of blood products in patients who need help.	Unnecessary and unsafe blood transfusions are dangerous. They can lead to severe responses or diseases caused by blood transfusions. Patients who need help may therefore have less access to blood donation.

6.8 Conclusion

The results show that enhanced translatability through pre-editing guided by predictive assessment has significantly reduced the rates of mistranslations in all four African languages. Setting the threshold at a low level such as 0.21 represents a conservative and effective approach to minimising the risk of false negative predictions after the revision process. This chapter shows that even with machine learning classifiers which are not perfect, or having imbalanced sensitivity and specificity pairs, which are more common in solving complex real-life issues, adjusting the probability threshold can still improve the usability, effectiveness of machine learning-based pre-editing assessment tools like ours. This novel approach has opened a new avenue in machine learning quality and reliability evaluation and improvement and has shown important research promise for closing the gap in health translation to minority, less-resourced languages, for which an urgent need of health translation quality assurance and lack of adequate staffing of translators and language service support remains a significant real-life challenge for people from these language and cultural communities around the world. This chapter developed machine learning classifiers which can predict the translatability of English environmental and health information into any of the four languages. In doing so, the predictive assessment tool developed can be applied in evaluating the quality of translations to these languages either individually or collectively. It presented a highly flexible and cost-effective approach to significantly boosting the confidence of developers of English health information intended for the purpose of community translation, engagement, education, and promotion. As the discussion above explained, the machine learning classifiers developed exhibited some limitations at this stage, which was reflected in the lack of balance of model sensitivity and specificity. This is however very common and realistic with the development of machine learning models using complex, real-life datasets, such as ours. As discussed in detail in the previous chapter, model accuracy does no translate readily into the model's practical usability. Since the African translation data that we collected exhibited greater irregularities and complexity, when compared to the Japanese translation readability datasets, the overall accuracy of the machine learning classifiers developed in this chapter was somewhat reduced, although was still over 70 per cent. To utilise the tool in real-life scenarios, which is to minimise the risk of false negative predictions following the revision of the English texts for translation use, we deliberately adjusted the threshold probability to a rather conservative level to ensure the safe use of the tool, and the reliability of the prediction outcome to guide the iterative improvement of the translatability of English texts into African minority languages.

CHAPTER 7

Assessing Linguistic Accessibility of Chinese Environmental and Health Information

7.1 Introduction

Much of current health translation research within the field of translation studies has focused on the quality of translations in terms of linguistic accuracy. However, the linguistic understandability and accessibility of health translation has been understudied. From the perspective of public health education, quality translations provide important resources for vulnerable populations with limited English proficiency, low general education or low health education levels, or other socio-economic determinants which can limit their access to first-hand, more complex health and medical information in English when compared with social groups and populations from more affluent socio-economic backgrounds.

In health and medical research, the term translation has been used extensively to describe the process of translating, adapting clinical or health research findings into practical social applications such as public health advice and health guidelines. By contrast, in translation studies, our primary focus of research is on the linguistic quality of translated health materials, products or services. In both fields, health translation evaluation is guided or perhaps more precisely, dominated by the views of experts: health or medical professionals in medical science, or translation scholars and language experts in translation studies.

The main social function of translations of public-oriented health and medical resources is however to inform, support, guide the decision making and health behaviours of individuals or populations in need. Given the complex nature of original health materials, it is argued that effective health translation should focus to deliver reliable health information of enhanced linguistic accessibility which reflects the general level of education of the intended readership. Improving the linguistic readability of translations of resources for the purpose of health education has important impact on the usability and communicative effectiveness of health translations. Effective health translations of increased understandability and actionability can help develop the health literacy of vulnerable social groups and help reduce their exposure to health risks and improve their self-health management abilities.

The recent outbreaks of the novel coronavirus around the world once again highlight the importance of developing linguistically accessible health translations for disadvantaged populations who have been affected most by the pandemic such as migrants, and people with varying cognitive and social vulnerabilities. Effective user-oriented health translations have formed an important layer of social protection.

Different from evaluation methods widely used in public health which require review and manual scoring of health translation understandability using clinically developed health information quality guidelines, translation researchers can work directly with health translations, and conduct multidimensional linguistic analyses of translated resources in comparison with original health resources in the target language. The rise and rapid growth of target-oriented descriptive translation studies over the last few decades has made important preparations for the development of empirical or statistical instruments to assess the linguistic comprehensibility of health materials translations between typologically different languages.

More recently, complex machine learning algorithms have been developed to enable rapid evaluation and prediction of the linguistic suitability and accessibility of English health materials for readers with specific needs or from different language and cultural backgrounds and with limited English proficiency. For example, Xie, Ji, & Hao (2021) developed, compared new machine learning algorithms, and their sensitivity, specificity, and accuracy in predicting the language accessibility of English health materials on infectious diseases for international tertiary students. The study collected first-hand materials from a range of English health websites and developed machine learning models to predict the easiness versus difficulty of original English health information among young adults from nonnative English-speaking backgrounds. The machine learning model which was developed revealed that while the difficulty of English health information can be explained by existing readability research, such as lexical unfamiliarity, medical terminology, and jargons, as well as syntactic complexity that can be measured by long and complex sentence structures, the easiness or understandability of original English material can be explained by more varied textual and semantic features including the use of common speech act verbs, familiar verbs of mental acts and processes, personal names and pronouns, names of social groups and communities, people's relations, expressions assisting with the evaluation of events, scenarios, or circumstances such as probability expressions, and expressions that direct or draw the attention of the readers to key points of the reading material such as adverbs describing levels, and degrees.

Limited research has been conducted to explore the linguistic accessibility of environmental and health information in Mandarin Chinese, which provides the focus of this corpus-based empirical study.

7.2 Methods

7.2.1 Data Collection

One of the key organisational responsibilities of the World Health Organization (WHO) is to provide objective, reliable information, and medical, health advice to the global public (WHO, 2005). WHO states that 'materials are issued or made accessible to the public ... for the purpose of communicating health knowledge and guidance' (WHO, 2016). To reach out to a culturally, linguistically diverse global audience, public-oriented health information from the WHO is translated to its official languages: French, Spanish, Arabic, Russian, and Chinese (WHO, 2017; Cronin, 2003; Toma, Guetterman, Yaqub, Talaat, & Fetters, 2017). Internationally, health information in Chinese developed by the WHO has an important impact on the acquisition of research-based health knowledge by the global Chinese-speaking readers (Wu, 1999). The China Centre of Disease Control (CCDC) is the national authority of health and medical research. It is the major source of Chinese health information for the Chinese public (Hipgrave, 2011; Xu, 1994; Cohen, Henderson, Aiello, & Zheng, 1996).

The website of the CCDC with its public-oriented structural design was adopted and launched to the public in mid-2005 (Li, 2004), focusing on increasing the wide accessibility and usability of health information beyond a narrowed target readership of medical and health professionals prior to 2005. An important structural reform of the CCDC website was its focus on providing authoritative health information and advice to inform, guide, and direct the Chinese public in the understanding and prevention of locally prevalent diseases and health risk factors. For example, in informing the public of the pandemic of human swine streptococcus disease, the CCDC website released health information on the investigation, monitoring, diagnosis, treatment of the pandemic, as well as knowledge of the pathogens, transmission routes, prevention and control. This represents an important ongoing effort by CCDC to align its public engagement strategies with international health authorities, especially the WHO. Public-oriented health information on the CCDC website is collected from national and local research centres which are affiliates of the CCDC; or not-for-profit organisations for health promotion (Appendix 7.1). However, the understandability or accessibility of these Chinese health resources among the Chinese-speaking public remain understudied. This study identified some persistent gaps between international and Chinese authorities in providing accessible information on infectious diseases to the Chinese public.

A comparable corpus was constructed which contained health texts of WHO and CCDC sources. Chinese health materials from the WHO were Chinese translations from original English materials and the Chinese materials from the CCDC were in original Chinese. Efforts were made to maintain the structural balance between the two sets of data and the collected health materials were allocated to folders on similar health topics broadly divided into infectious diseases, antibiotics, accidents, disability, pregnancy and maternity, environmental health, non-communicable diseases (diabetes, cancers, cardiovascular diseases, etc.), mental health, capacity building, dementia, and tobacco control. Some topics were well represented in both sources of Chinese health information such as infectious diseases, pregnancy and maternity, environmental health, non-communicable diseases, and some topics were absent from the CCDC website such as mental health, dementia, antibiotics, capacity building, and accidents. This was partly due to the global reach of the WHO and the diversity of health topics covered by the international health organisation, and partly due to the lack of relevant health educational materials on topics such as mental health, dementia, and disability from the Chinese health authority. The total number of individual health texts collected for the corpus was close to 1000 with a balanced divide between the two sources (see Appendix 7.1).

7.2.2 *Measuring the Readability of Health Materials*

The readability of health resources can be assessed using readability formulas (See Table 7.1). With English, there are a variety of tools for readability research (Flesch, 1948; Gunning, 1952; Coleman & Liau, 1975; McLaughlin, 1969; Senter & Smith, 1967; O'Hayre, 1966). Some of the key features used for assessing health information readability are lexical familiarity, cognitive complexity, and morphological complexity.

These can be measured by quantifiable textual and linguistic features such as average sentence length, average number of syllables per word, percentage of hard words, average number of words in sentences, and so

Table 7.1 *Readability formulas*

Readability Tools	Formula
Flesch Reading Ease Score	Score = 206.835–(1.015*ASL[a]) – (84.6*ASW[b])
Gunning Fog	Score = 0.4*(ASL[a]+PHW[c])
Flesch-Kincaid Grade Level	Score = (0.39 * ASL[a]) + (11.8*ASW[b])–15.59
Coleman-Liau Index	Score = 5.89*ACW[d]–0.3*sentence/(100*words)–15.8
SMOG Index	Score = 3 + Square Root of Polysyllable Count
Automated Readability Index	Score = (AVL[e]*4.71) +(AVW[f]*0.5)–21.43
Linsear Write Formula	Score = (Easy words*1+Hard words*3)/Sentence count If >20, divided by '2'; If <20 or =20, subtract '2', and divide by '2'.

[a] ASL: average sentence length; [b] ASW: average number of syllables per word; [c] PHW: percentage of hard words; [d] ACW: average character per word; [e] AVL: average number of letters per word; [f] AVW: average number of words in sentences

on. Some of the widely used English readability tools include Flesch Reading Ease, Gunning Fog, Flesch-Kincaid Grade Level, Coleman-Liau Index, SMOG Index, Automated Readability Index and Linsear Write Formula. Despite reported inconsistency among these readability tools, they are still widely regarded as convenient methods for a rapid diagnosis of the understandability of health resources for populations from different educational backgrounds.

Chinese is distinct from languages which use the Latin alphabet. Structural adjustment is required to develop empirical instruments to assess the understandability of health information written in Chinese. In this study of the complexity of health information in original and translated Chinese, the Chinese Readability Index Explorer (CRIE) was used which was developed by the National Taiwan Normal University (Sung, Chang, & Lin, 2016; Yan et al., 2021; Yu-Ta, Yaw-Huei, and Yu-Chih, 2013). CRIE enables high-dimensional, integrated linguistic analyses of Chinese texts, and ranks their readability (for Chinese readers from Grade 1 to 8 educational backgrounds) according to the assessment score of individual linguistic items. In this study, features of CRIE which were directly relevant to health text readability evaluation were selected to measure the lexical difficulty, semantic complexity, and orthographic complexity of Chinese characters, and the level of information load of health information in Chinese as described below.

It should be noted that the CRIE system was originally developed to evaluate traditional Chinese or Fantizi used in Taiwan. In mainland China, the standard written form of Chinese is simplified Chinese or

Jiantizi. Fantizi is orthographically much more complex than Jiantizi, as the average number of strokes per Fantizi is significantly higher than Jiantizi. As a result, in measuring the orthographic complexity of health information developed by CCDC and the WHO which are all in Jiantizi, the more neutral linguistic feature 'average stroke per character' was chosen, instead of features such as low-stroke (with total strokes between one to ten), middle-stroke (eleven to twenty), or high-stroke (over twenty-one strokes) characters as defined by the CRIE system.

7.2.3 Lexical Difficulty

Lexical difficulty was measured by the ratio between difficult Chinese words and the total number of words of the articles we collected from the WHO and CCDC websites, respectively. Sung et al. (2016) discussed the selection criteria for Chinese difficult words. They first created a word frequency list for the balanced corpus used in their study (CKIP, 1998). Then they used the first 3,000 words to create a 'commonly used words' list. Words that did not appear in this list were designated as difficult words, which in turn were used to develop the difficult words feature of the CRIE system. In this study, a large variety of health texts were collected covering topics such as capacity building (WHO only), accidents (WHO only), disability (WHO only), non-communicable diseases (both WHO and CCDC), mental health (WHO only), pregnancy and maternity (both WHO and CCDC), dementia (WHO only), tobacco control (both WHO and CCDC), environmental health (both WHO and CCDC), nutrition (both WHO and CCDC), antibiotic (WHO) and infectious diseases (WHO and CCDC). As an international health organisation, WHO covers a much broader range of health topics than CCDC.

7.2.4 Semantic Complexity

Semantic complexity was measured using the ratio between sentences of complex semantic expressions (polysemous words) and the total number of sentences in the Chinese health materials. Sung et al. (2016) noted that polysemous words are often the most difficult to deal with in the development of the CRIE system, but they are also the most important linguistic feature. Since polysemous words have relatively complex semantic structures, they are more likely to introduce discrepancies. Because words with several meanings have more semantic categories, the developers of the CRIE system used semantic categorisation to determine the degree of complexity of polysemes.

Polysemy is also an important linguistic phenomenon in health linguistics. Usual or common words can have distinct meanings when used in specialised health and medical domains. For example, the word 'culture', when used in common, everyday language, means 'The way of life of a people, including their attitudes, values, beliefs, arts, sciences, modes of perception, and habits of thought and activity'. However, when used in microbiology, the word culture means 'the propagation of microorganisms in a growth medium. Any body tissue or fluid can be evaluated in the laboratory by using culture techniques to detect and identify infectious processes.' This is a typical example of polysemous words which can increase the semantic complexity of health materials.

In modern Chinese, the possibility of polysemous verbs is much higher than that of nouns and adjectives. According to the statistics of the corpus of primary and secondary school textbooks, the frequency of verbs accounts for 44 per cent of the total frequency of Chinese content words, while the frequency of polysemous verbs accounts for 59 per cent of the total frequency of polysemous content words, polysemous nouns account for 22 per cent, and polysemous adjectives for 13 per cent. There are numerous examples of polysemous words in written materials. For example, the character 想 (Xiǎng) can be translated as want, think, wish, suppose, believe, miss, feel like doing, would like, etc. The character 气 Qì can be interpreted as gas, air, breath, spirit, weather, odour, vital energy, gaseous, etc. The character 安 (Ān) can mean safe, secure, quiet, calm, content, satisfied, still, install, fit, pacify, fix. Despite the increase of bi- or tri-character words in modern Chinese, compared to the predominance of mono-character words in classical Chinese which are more likely to be polysemous, polysemy is still a distinct feature of Chinese writing. Bi-character words like 出入 Chūrù can be translated as entrance and exit, inconsistent, go out and come in, expenditure and income, or discrepancy.

Appendix 7.2 gives some typical examples of polysemous words in Mandarin Chinese.

7.2.5 *Orthographic Complexity*

Chinese is a distinct language from languages which use the Latin alphabet. The basic orthographic unit of Chinese script is a stroke rather than a syllable. In China, there are two different ways of writing Chinese characters. One is called simplified Chinese, which was made to make it easier for people to learn. The other way is called traditional Chinese, which is the older way of writing. Most Chinese-speaking places like China, Singapore, and Malaysia use a simpler way of writing characters, while Hong Kong and Taiwan still use the traditional way. Some characters were made simpler, but not all of them. Around half of the most used characters were changed to be easier to write, with fewer strokes, while the remaining stayed the same in both simplified and traditional Chinese script. There were debates around the introduction of simplified characters. Some believed that simplified characters made it easier for ordinary people to learn and acquire knowledge, but others argued that just reducing the number of strokes might make them harder to learn at a later stage. That is because, when a person increases their lexical reserve, simplified characters might start to look less distinguishable. Research has shown that the perception of the orthographic complexity of the Chinese script is highly related to one's cultural and educational backgrounds. For Chinese people familiar with the traditional character form and with higher educational levels, orthographic complexity does not necessarily present a reading and comprehension challenge. In this study, we still use orthography as a contributing factor to the comprehension of Chinese written health information in line with existing research in the field. Current readability tools mostly evaluate the orthographic complexity of English or European languages using measurements such as average number of syllables per word. In this study of the orthographic complexity of Chinese characters, we used the average stroke per Chinese character as the measurement, which can be obtained by dividing the total number of strokes in a certain text by the total number of individual characters as a basic unit of Chinese written script See Table 7.2.

7.2.6 Lexical Density

Information load has been studied extensively in the evaluation of the readability of health information. In this study, information load was assessed using the measurement of the density of content words in Chinese health information. Content words include a variety of Chinese words such as nouns, verbs, adjectives, and adverbs. Their main function in a health text is to indicate objectives, actions, processes, agents of health and medical activities. The density of content words refers to the ratio of content words and the total number of words in a Chinese health text. It was noted in the Chinese corpus analysis that complex lexis such as technical terms (TT), proper nouns (PN), names of diseases and chemicals (NA) made up the bulk of the health texts collected. Examples in Appendix 7.3 illustrate the importance of lexical density for Chinese readers to process and comprehend environmental and health information, either in original Chinese or in translated Chinese.

Table 7.2 *Distribution of strokes among the most common 7,000 characters in Mandarin Chinese*

Stroke number	Number of the most common 7,000 characters	Percentage
1	3	0.04
2	22	0.31
3	63	0.90
4	137	1.96
5	203	2.90
6	362	5.17
7	566	8.09
8	710	10.14
9	780	11.14
10	768	10.97
11	732	10.46
12	688	9.83
13	552	7.89
14	418	5.97
15	340	4.86
16	265	3.79
17	192	2.74
18	93	1.26
19	88	0.97
20	68	0.39
21	27	0.29
22	20	0.23
23	16	0.11
24	8	0.10
25	7	0.01
26	1	0.01
28	1	0.01
30	1	0.00

7.3 Comparison of Health Information Complexity from the China Centre of Disease Control and the World Health Organization

7.3.1 *Comparing Lexical Difficulty*

Table 7.3 shows the Mann-Whitney U Test comparing Chinese health information on six large health topics from the WHO and CCDC sources. Statistically significant differences were found between the two sets of health texts on environmental health ($p=0.011$, $r=0.284$) and infectious diseases

Table 7.3 *Mann-Whitney U Test (ratio of difficult words)*

Topics	WHO (I) – CCDC (J) Mean Difference (I-J)	Sig. (2-tailed) (p)	Effect Size (r)
Environmental health	−0.0457	0.011 **	0.2839
Infectious diseases	−0.0380	0.000 **	0.2504
Pregnancy and maternity	−0.0961	0.001 **	0.6074
Non-communicable diseases	0.0041	0.965	0.0090
Nutrition	−0.0601	0.131	0.2716
Tobacco control	−0.0066	0.602	0.1651

Table 7.4 *Mann-Whitney U Test (ratio of sentences of complex semantics (polysemous words)*

Topics	WHO (I) – CCDC (J) Mean Difference (I-J)	Sig. (2-tailed) (p)	Effect Size (r)
Environmental health	−0.090758	0.007 **	0.2971
Infectious diseases	−0.071250	0.000 **	0.2373
Pregnancy and maternity	−0.114859	0.068	0.3328
Non-communicable diseases	−0.029762	0.827	0.045
Nutrition	−0.054709	0.522	0.1150
Tobacco control	−0.125474	0.209	0.3975

(p=0.00, r= 0.2504). Chinese health information from the CCDC on pregnancy and maternity care was lexically more difficult than Chinese health information from the WHO (p=0.001, r=0.6074). By contrast, differences in lexical difficulty between WHO and CCDC in covering other health topics such as non-communicable diseases (p=0.965), nutrition (p=0.131) and tobacco control (p=0.602) were not statistically significant.

7.3.2 Comparing Cognitive Complexity

Table 7.4 shows that the Mann Whitney U Test of two sets of health texts from the WHO and CCDC. It shows that like Table 7.1, statistically significant differences were found between WHO and CCDC health information in covering health topics of environmental health (p=0.007, r=0.2971) and infectious diseases (p=0.00, r=0.2373). By contrast, the distribution of sentences of complex semantic meanings, that is, the rate

Table 7.5 *Mann-Whitney U Test (average strokes per character)*

Topics	WHO (I) – CCDC (J) Mean Difference (I-J)	Sig. (2-tailed) (p)	Effect Size (r)
Environmental health	−0.118617	0.133	0.1669
Infectious diseases	−0.077977	0.004 **	0.1636
Pregnancy and maternity	−0.317984	0.023 **	0.4165
Non-communicable diseases	0.413108	0.239	0.2405
Nutrition	−0.132644	0.171	0.2461
Tobacco control	−0.094873	0.602	0.1651

of use of polysemous words was largely similar between WHO and CCDC health information in covering topics such as pregnancy and maternity (p=0.068), non-communicable diseases (p=0.827), nutrition (p=0.522) and tobacco control (p=0.209).

7.3.3 *Comparing Orthographic Complexity*

Table 7.5 shows that in the Mann-Whitney U Test, statistically significant differences in the orthographic depth of health texts were found between WHO and CCDC health information covering infectious diseases (p=0.133, r = 0.1669) and pregnancy and maternity (p=0.004, 0.1636). Differences between WHO and CCDC in the use of orthographically complex words when covering health topics such as environmental health (p=0.133), non-communicable diseases (p=0.239), nutrition (p=0.171), tobacco control (p=0.602) were however statistically insignificant.

7.3.4 *Information Load*

Table 7.6 shows that statistically significant differences were found between WHO and CCDC information in terms of their information load when covering health topics such as environmental health (p=0.000, r=0.5122) and infectious diseases (p=0.000, r=0.2937). By contrast, there were no statistically significant differences between WHO and CCDC resources in terms of information load when covering health topics of pregnancy and maternity care (p=0.630), non-communicable diseases (p=0.760), nutrition (p=0.080) and tobacco control (p=0.917). The higher levels of information load of Chinese health texts on environmental health and infectious diseases resemble the finding on the higher semantic complexity of these two types of Chinese

Table 7.6 *Mann-Whitney U Test (density of content words)*

Topics	WHO (I) – CCDC (J) Mean Difference (I-J)	Sig. (2-tailed) (p)	Effect Size (r)
Environmental health	−0.03694	0.000 **	0.5122
Infectious diseases	−0.02127	0.000**	0.2937
Pregnancy and maternity	−0.000568	0.630	0.0878
Non-communicable diseases	−0.00499	0.760	0.0625
Nutrition	−0.02179	0.080	0.3140
Tobacco control	−0.00696	0.917	0.033

Table 7.7 *Dimensions of Chinese health information complexity*

Dimensions	Measurement	Average Level of Chinese Health Resources from WHO
Lexical Difficulty	Ratio of difficult words	0.3619
Cognitive Complexity	Ratio of complex semantics	0.4334
Orthographic Complexity	Average strokes per character	7.7255
Information Load	Density of content words	0.8218
SIUCHI Index Reference		0.33565

health texts from CCDC, suggesting that environmental health and infectious diseases from CCDC are the two varieties of Chinese health texts of the highest complexity in terms of semantic complexity and information load of health information.

Table 7.7 shows the various dimensions of Chinese health information complexity. The index contains the four dimensions discussed above. The reference value of each dimension was based on the mean of the average values for each dimension of assessment of Chinese health texts from the WHO on a balanced range of topics of public health information: nutrition, disability, pregnancy and maternity care, environmental health, infectious diseases, non-communicable diseases, and mental health.

7.4 Receiver Operating Characteristic Analysis

Receiver Operating Characteristic (ROC) Curve Analysis is widely used in clinical research to assess the diagnostic ability of health and medical research tools, for example, the prediction of the existence of diseases or medical conditions in a patient. In this study, a ROC analysis was conducted to evaluate the prediction of Chinese health materials from either WHO or China CDC sources. The predictor variables were the four separate evaluation parameters: the Density of content words, Ratio of Difficult Words, Average Strokes per character, Ratio of sentences with complex semantic categories, and the Chinese health information complexity Index (CHICI). The positive actual state was CCDC, and the negative actual state was the WHO. Sensitivity was associated with the model's ability to predict health information from the CCDC sources; whereas specificity was associated with the model's ability to precisely predict health information from the WHO sources.

Table 7.8 compares the performance of the five diagnostic instruments to predict the origin of Chinese health information from either CCDC or WHO, using the four separate accessibility evaluation dimensions and the compound index as predictors, respectively. The Area under the Curve (AUC) measures the overall performance of the tools. It shows the index instrument achieved the highest AUC of 0.716 with 95 per cent Confidence Intervals (CI) of 0.673 and 0.759. This is statistically higher than the AUC (0.5) of the null hypothesis, indicating that the instrument can be used effectively to discriminate health texts from WHO or CCDC sources. The instruments based on the four evaluation parameters had also achieved statistically higher AUCs than the null hypothesis. The instrument using the Ratio of Difficult Words (lexical complexity) as the discriminating feature achieved the second highest AUC of 0.691 (95 per cent CI: 0.647, 0.735). This was followed by the diagnostic instrument using Density of Content Words (information load) which achieved an AUC of 0.672 (95 per cent CI: 0.624, 0.72). A less effective diagnostic tool was the one measuring semantic complexity (Ratio of Sentences with complex semantic categories) which achieved an AUC of 0.650 (95 per cent CI: 0.602, 0.697). The least effective tool was the one which discriminated health text sources using orthographic complexity of texts (Average Strokes per character) which obtained a mean AUC of 0.636 (95 per cent CI: 0.589, 0.683). This finding suggests that the order of linguistic features which can be used to distinguish health texts from the two sources of information were lexical difficulty, information load, semantic complexity (polysemy which requires specialised health domain knowledge) and orthographic complexity.

Appendix 7.4 shows the results of the paired-sample t test of the five diagnostic tools. It shows that statistically significant improvements were achieved from the orthographic complexity model to the lexical complexity

Table 7.8 *Area under the receiver operating characteristic curve*

				Asymptotic 95% Confidence Interval	
Test Result Variable(s)	Area under the Curve	Std. Error[a]	Asymptotic Sig.[b]	Lower Bound	Upper Bound
Simple index of the linguistic understandability of Chinese health information (SIUCHI)	0.716	0.022	0.000	0.673	0.759
Ratio of Difficult Words (DWRatio)	0.691	0.022	0.000	0.647	0.735
Density of content words	0.672	0.024	0.000	0.624	0.720
Ratio of sentences with complex semantic categories	0.650	0.024	0.000	0.602	0.697
Average Strokes per character	0.636	0.024	0.000	0.589	0.683

a. Under the nonparametric assumption. The analysis was conducted using SPSS version 21.
b. Null hypothesis: true area = 0.5

model (p=0.020); from the orthographic complexity model to the index-based model (p=0.000); from the semantic complexity model to the index-based model (p=0.018); and from the orthographic complexity model to the index-based model pair (p=0.000).

7.5 Conclusion

For the CCDC, our study found that Chinese health information from the CCDC on infectious diseases is more complex and difficult to understand than Chinese health information on similar topics from the WHO. This was evidenced in the statistically greater lexical difficulty, higher semantic complexity, deeper orthographic depth, and higher information load of health information on infectious diseases from CCDC sources, when compared to Chinese health information from the WHO. This study demonstrates that important improvements need to be made urgently to close persistent gaps in the understandability of Chinese health resources developed by the CCDC, as our study shows that they are statistically more complex, difficult to understand than Chinese health information developed by the WHO aimed at a global Chinese-speaking public. For the WHO, although Chinese health information on infectious diseases from the WHO were largely at the average level of all health topics, in terms of semantic complexity, orthographic depth and information load, the use of difficult Chinese words in health information from WHO was however higher than the average level, indicating the need to address the lexical complexity issue in the development of Chinese language resources at the WHO, especially when the resources are aimed at the general Chinese-speaking public.

Improving the accessibility of health information can have important, transgenerational impact on the health literacy of the Chinese public. Accessible health information can not only help the public to prevent infectious diseases more effectively, but also help improve the health and wellbeing of vulnerable populations such as women, children and those exposed to greater risks of environmental health issues such as air and water pollution. This study shows that infectious diseases, pregnancy and maternity care and environmental health are the least accessible or most difficult-to-understand areas and topics of Chinese health information. Accessibility of public-oriented health information in Chinese remains understudied. There is an urgent need to address the lack of accessibility to critical health information for Chinese readers. The WHO has an important role in leading the efforts to improve the accessibility of global authoritative health resources in local languages. National authorities have the responsibility to develop locally relevant and more accessible health information on infectious diseases, as improving accessible health knowledge represents a most effective health policy to reduce health risks.

This study has a limitation that can be improved in future work on health information accessibility. First, the simplified index of the understandability of Chinese health information (SIUCHI) was designed to provide a rapid, convenient evaluation of the difficulty of health texts for readers using simplified Chinese in mainland China. For readers among other Chinese communities using traditional Chinese script, the tool needs further adjustment. For example, although orthographic complexity or high-stroke character words can cause significant reading difficulties for readers using simplified Chinese or Jiantizi, higher orthographic complexity can greatly facilitate the reading of Chinese written materials among readers using the Fantizi system such as residents in Taiwan, Hong Kong, and many migrant Chinese communities in English-speaking countries. Second, in this study, Chinese health information developed by the WHO was used as reference material or the benchmark of comparison for information complexity. Research and policy documents however have reported that improvement is needed to ensure the wider accessibility of WHO resources (Carter, 2005; Carter, 1999; Nasser et al., 2015; WHO, 2008; Doherty et al., 2015), and the WHO is currently engaged in the assessment of the global social impact of their publications beyond policy makers and health professionals (Ennis, McKay, Ly, Dyke, Deonandan, 2015). Research is needed for the assessment of the local language versions of WHO resources intended for culturally and linguistically diverse global readerships.

This study shows that both the WHO and national health authorities like the CCDC have an important responsibility to increase the linguistic accessibility of authoritative health information among the public, such as those on critical health topics such as infectious diseases, environmental health, pregnancy and maternity, mental health, and disability. Improving the linguistic accessibility of this information can help improve health literacy and health information equality. This is essential to help achieve the United Nations sustainable development goal (SDG) on universal healthcare and health information accessibility for vulnerable populations.

CHAPTER 8

Conclusion

Buse and Weimer (2008) define 'readability' as a human judgement of how easy a text is to understand. Over the years, a great number of quantitative measures of readability have been developed, and these are the focus of this book. In Chapter 1 we traced the history of readability measures, from the traditional formulas of the mid-twentieth century to the machine learning models of today. Chapter 2 looked at the statistical techniques which are used in the remainder of the book, and includes sections on the machine learning techniques of Logistic Regression (LR) and Support Vector Machines (SVM) which are used by Meng Ji in her experiments described in Chapters 3 to 6. While Chapters 1 and 2 considered traditional uses of readability measures to gauge how hard or easy a text is to read, Chapters 3 to 6 took a much more novel approach. Chapters 3 and 4 considered the readability of texts in the field of health education, but this information is taken not as an end in itself, but to predict whether the texts are more suitable for a general readership or a more specific readership, the parents and caregivers of young children. Chapter 5 used the readability scores obtained for English texts on the environment to predict whether these texts will be translated into readable Japanese. Finally, Chapter 6 used the readability scores for environmental texts to predict whether the texts can be accurately machine translated. This is tested by translating the texts into four African languages with Google Translate, then translating them back with Microsoft Bing Translate, to see whether any errors appear during this two-way process. Meng Ji wrote Chapters 3, 4, 5, 6 and 7 while Michael Oakes wrote Chapters 1 and 2, and this conclusion.

Chapter 1 introduced previous research on readability measures. Traditional readability measures look at easy-to-measure features of text such as word length, number of syllables per word and number of complex words from a list. Many early measures used a combination of these features to predict the Grade Point Level, the school year in the United States Education System in which the average student would be able to read a text comfortably. Early readability measures used multiple regression (see Section 2.7) to relate the predictor variables to the outcome variable of readability score. The readability of a text could be estimated independently using a version of the Cloze test. Later work made use of psychological theory and considered such things as coherence, density and information load. More recently, advances in Natural Language Processing (NLP) have enabled the use of syntactic parsing, statistical language modelling, and machine learning which creates automatic classifiers. The standard corpora (large collections of text stored electronically for language research) which have been used in machine learning for readability are described just after the section on machine learning itself. Next, we looked at techniques which come under the umbrella term of language models, a very topical notion as they include ChatGPT. We then considered another class of machine learning models called deep learning, an extension of neural networks. The first language for which readability measures were developed was English, but we also look at more recent work on Italian, Swedish, French, German, and Indian languages.

Chapter 2 introduced basic statistics and machine learning for readability measures. In this short introduction to statistics, we looked closely at some statistics which have been used in the development of readability measures. Data sets are often characterised by their 'average' value and the degree of variability of the data, and we looked at both these concepts. We examined the 'bell curve' typical of normally distributed statistical data, and its relation to hypothesis testing. The Mann-Whitney Test is described to answer the question of whether the type-token ratio is greater in high or low readability texts. Simple regression using Pearson's product moment correlation test is described with the example of answering the question of to what extent does the readability score vary with the number of unique monosyllables in a text? We then moved onto multiple regression, where the variation of the readability score is viewed as a function of four predictor variables: number of words, type-token ratio, syllables per word and the number of proper nouns. The selection of which variables really do have an effect on readability can be made in two ways: it can be assigned a statistically significant p-value, or we can use Akaike's Information Criterion. Logistic regression can be considered as both a traditional statistical test or as a method of machine learning. We also considered the other machine learning technique used widely in the experiments described in Chapters 3 to 6, namely Support Vector Machines.

Chapter 3 explored the readability of environmental health resources for parental education. Communicating environmental health risks is a challenging and sometimes daunting research topic. In order to achieve better health promotion outcomes for diverse groups of people with varying levels of reading skill, there is a need for better, targeted, understandable and effective communication to render it more inclusive (Lundgren & McMakin, 2013). The World Health Organization (WHO) Strategic Communication Framework desiderata for effective health communications are that a text should be accessible (available through various media such as printed texts, internet and radio), actionable (are the recommendations practical to carry out?), credible (accurate, clear and consistent), relevant (suitable for specific populations), timely (making sure that information does not arrive too late, such as making sure that flood prevention advice does not arrive after the flood has occurred), and understandable (comprehensible to the intended readership, including those without relevant technical expertise). Readability is a prerequisite to understanding, which itself is a prerequisite to achieving relevance, credibility and actionability. This chapter examined the applicability and limitations of quantitative readability tools in predicting the likely readership of online environmental health education resources.

In the first experiment, four traditional readability metrics (Flesch Reading Ease, SMOG, FORCAST and Gunning Fog) were used as binary classifiers to predict the suitability of health-related texts for either the general public or specific readerships such as the parents of young children. The four traditional reading metrics were compared by specificity (the ratio of correct positive assignments to all positive assignments) and sensitivity (the ratio of the number of articles correctly classified by the measure as negative to all articles judged negative). Here 'negative' might refer to articles classified as being 'for parents', when 'positive' would refer to articles classified as being 'for the public'. For each measure, a Receiver-Operator (ROC) curve was produced, which is a graph of 1–Specificity on the x axis and Sensitivity on the y axis. The measure which produces the curve highest above the diagonal (where 1-Specificity and Sensitivity are equal) is taken to be the best classifier, in this case Flesh Reading Ease. To choose the optimal cut-off point whereby any article with a higher readability would be assigned to the parents class (or otherwise to the public class), a value resulting in the specificity and sensitivity both being above the arbitrary threshold of 0.7 was chosen. For the Flesch Reading Ease measure, the optimal cut-off point was in the range 42.5 to 44.5.

Construction of the corpus of environmental materials was achieved with just over a million words in each section of the corpus. As examples of the sources, Healthline Media, Centers for Disease Control and Prevention, the

Mayo Clinic, and the National Institute of Environmental Health Sciences were used in the building of the public corpus. The parents' corpus included texts from the New Zealand Dermatological Society, Cancer Council Australia, Centers for Disease Control and Prevention, Emergency Response, and the World Health Organization. A topic model created using the technique of Latent Dirichlet Analysis showed that the composition of the two sub-corpora was very similar. The topic modelling produced a list of keywords most typical of the discovered topics, and it was found that topics 0 (water safety) and 8 (skin conditions) were predominant in both sub-corpora. Thus we were confident that there was no significant thematic variation between the two sub-corpora.

The four binary classifiers used Flesch Reading Ease, SMOG, FORCAST and the Gunning Fog Index as predictors, respectively. But these classifiers had imbalanced sensitivity and specificity scores, which was the main reason we developed machine learning classifiers (described in Chapter 4) which had both higher sensitivity and specificity scores. The main advantage of assessing articles automatically according to the desired readership is greater convenience and cost-effectiveness. Chapter 4 used machine learning to identify new linguistic features (at higher levels than the length of words and sentences) to predict the suitability of environmental texts for either the general public or the parents or caregivers of young children, an example of a general and a specific readership respectively.

Chapter 4 explored the suitability of environmental health information for parental education using machine learning models. Statistics were used to determine whether environmental health texts were more suitable for the general public or for the parents of young children. In general, this provides a method to facilitate the production for targeted audiences. The resulting multiple logistic regression model provides linguistically interpretable results. Performing this task using readability formulas which are based on such superficial features as word length and sentence length is not accurate enough. The aims of using Machine Learning were first to increase the accuracy of the classifiers, and second to consider individual differences between readers rather than using a 'one size fits all' formula. Actually, we do not quite consider differences at the level of every individual, but we do consider two groups of readers: the general public and the parents and caregivers of young children. Both groups are considered to be homogeneous, with the parents being assumed to have a Year 10 education and to come from an English-speaking background.

As well as considering surface linguistic features (which traditional measures do), we also looked to see the effect of semantic, sentiment, lexico-grammatical and syntactic factors. Studies of these features was enabled by corpus feature annotation. UCREL Semantic Analysis System (USAS) (Rayson Archer, Piao, & McEnery, 2004) gives each relevant word in the text a semantic code such as the main discourse headers arts and crafts, the body and the individual, housing, money and sports and games. Altogether we used all twenty-one main headers as possible semantic codes. SEANCE (Szkody & McKinney, 2022) tags each emotion-related word, such as words for anger, anxiety, boredom and contempt. Readability Studio (Shedlosky-Shoemaker, Sturm, Saleem, & Kelly, 2009) tags the text with a variety of lexical, grammatical and syntactic features such as the number of difficult sentences containing more than twenty-two words) and the number of characters including punctuation. Such features are more like those used in traditional measures of readability, but others give deeper annotation, such as the passive voice. There is some overlap in these three feature sets, as they were developed independently of each other. The total number of features would be too large to handle and result in a less generalisable model, so feature reduction was performed using a procedure called recursive feature elimination. In particular, this reduced the number of overlapping features. A Support Vector Machine was used as the basis for recursive feature elimination for automated feature optimisation, and a Logistic Regression-based classifier was developed for prediction of whether a text was more suitable for the general public or parents. The cross-validation was conducted on the training set, which was 70 per cent of the total data collected. We then used the cross-validated Machine Learning classifier to predict the remaining 30 per cent of the dataset, and observed whether the Machine Learning prediction was the same as the human evaluation of the machine translation output. We retained the features which minimised the cross-validation error.

Overall, recursive feature elimination cut the number of linguistic features from 390 to 65. In the corpus, there were 963 articles designed for the public, and 1133 articles designed for parents. Machine learning was by logistic regression, using 70 per cent training and 30 per cent testing data, with the parents' texts labelled 1 and the public texts 0. The resulting models had high sensitivity and specificity.

In order to rationalise the model, statistical feature selection (to cut down the number of features yet further) was done by the Mann-Whitney Test. The method was to check the effect size, which is a measure of the difference in type-token ratio values in the high and low readability groups. It is related to the z-score derived in the hand-calculated example of Chapter 2, and is given by the expression $r = z / \sqrt{N}$, where r is the effect size, z is the z-score and N is the sample size (Field, 2000: 227). The two criteria used to retain a feature were both that it produced a p-value below 0.001 and the effect size was greater than 0.1. Features more typical of public texts were associated with a language style that was analytical (containing abstract terms relating to the level of safety or danger), formal (such as 'wordy' items), moral or ethical (assessment of moral disapproval or misfortune), emphatic (overused words) or complex (such as the number of words with more than six characters, misspellings or out-of-dictionary words). Features more typical of a communicative style directed towards parents were supportive (words of affiliation or supportiveness), informal (casual or slang words), emotional (such as verbs of mental or emotional states), interactive (words referring to children) or instructive (human behaviour patterns). Overall, the features more typical of articles suitable for the public are interrelated, and indicate a higher-level, less engaging communication style than those for parents. With a small number of modifications (the removal of overlapping features and the addition of second person pronouns, emotions of fear and words of comparison) the final model (RF16) was produced. It had the advantages of parsimony (with only sixteen features) and being linguistically interpretable.

A multiple logistic regression was performed on the refined model of sixteen features, and for each feature a value Exp(B) was given, which was the odds ratio between texts geared for parents and those suitable for the general public. Coefficients greater than 1 meant that the value of a feature suggested the text was more suitable for the public, and lower values meant that the value of this feature was more typical of texts for parents. Abstract terms related to the level of safety or danger, and words of comparison, wordy items, words related to government and number of complex or misspelt words were predictors of texts for the general public. These words were more typical of analytical language. Conversely, the language of texts more suitable for parents included words of affiliation or supportiveness.

Assessment of the readability of environmental information is intrinsically linked with the unique linguistic and textual features of a language and culture. Environmental information accessible in one language may prove inaccessible in another language, as the definition and quantification of readability varies across languages and cultures. Chapter 5 explored the quantitative relationship between the complexity of English source texts of natural disasters and the readability of their translations in the Japanese language. The main purpose of Chapter 5 is to first, explore the impact of English linguistic and textual features on the readability of Japanese translations. Second, we leverage machine learning techniques to predict and improve the readability of Japanese translations through an informed and optimal design of English information on natural disasters and environmental health risks such as air, water and soil pollution, radiation, and exposure to harmful chemicals. The key results include machine learning models which are characterised by their linguistic interpretability, structural simplicity, and usefulness for improving the accessibility of natural disaster and emergency information in English-speaking multicultural countries.

Chapter 5 considered the effect of the linguistic features of an English text on its translation into Japanese. As an example, we looked at texts in the domain of natural disasters caused by extreme adverse weather conditions. 'Translation for educational purposes requires tailoring the translation to increase its understandability, trustworthiness and cultural affinity for the reader' (Ji & Sörenson, 2020). Here we looked at tailoring the source text (English) to improve the target text of Japanese. To illustrate, we described the development of machine learning classifiers (Support Vector Machines) for the prediction of whether an English text would be translated into accessible language. We used Japanese as a case study because of the linguistic and cultural contrast between English and Japanese. To build the corpus we used English-language web pages such as 'Bushfires and your health', 'Do facemasks protect you from bushfire smoke' and 'Burns and scalds'. Linguistic feature annotation of the texts was done by Readability Studio and USAS. The readability of Japanese texts can be measured on a scale devised by Jaeho Lee, as described in Chapter 5. Texts can be classified into one of six levels, but the cut-off point of interest to us is that texts with scores greater than 2.5 were considered readable in our experiments, and scores below 2.5 were taken to indicate texts with low readability. According to the scale, low readability texts would only be accessible to people who 'can understand most specialised texts, and can understand complex structures found in literary and other works'.

A Logistic Regression (LR) analysis was performed to show the impact of six linguistic features of the English texts on the readability of their Japanese translations. We compared linear SVM and radial basis function kernel (RBF) SVM for automated feature (see Chapter 5, Table 5.5) and decided to use linear SVM with six English source text features as the final model (Chapter 5, Table 5.3). We first used LR to identify English linguistic features which were significantly associated with the binary outcome, i.e. whether the Japanese translation is readable or not. We did this to solve the problem that machine learning selected features often are statistically significantly associated with the prediction outcome, adding to the difficulty of interpreting the machine learning models, and guide practical translation quality improvement. The use of proper nouns and punctuation can increase the readability of translations. The increased use of adpositions (prepositions and postpositions such as under, towards, and before, used to indicate the relationships between nouns in a sentence), increases its complexity. Not surprisingly, higher scores on three traditional readability measures (Flesch-Kincaid, Danielson-Bryan 1 and Coleman-Liau, where a higher score means a higher grade point level required to read the text) were associated with less readable translations.

Support Vector Machines (SVM) were constructed using these six linguistic features, the best of which according to the ROC curve method was a linear SVM with z-score normalisation. The SVM was used to classify English texts into those with a probability of more than 0.5 of producing 'safe' or 'risky' Japanese texts according to whether they were more likely to produce readable or non-readable Japanese translations. This enabled the likelihood of the text being translated into high or low readability Japanese to be calculated before the text is translated, and can be done by someone who is a domain expert in disaster information but not necessarily fluent in Japanese. If the posterior probability is more than 0.43, as is the case in Chapter 5, Figure 5.4, the text should be simplified by increasing the number of punctuation marks and proper nouns, or lowering the Grade level scores from the Danielson-Bryan 1 (reducing the number of characters in a word), Flesch-Kincaid (increasing the total number of words but reducing the number of syllables in a word) and Coleman-Liau (reducing the number of sentences). In Chapter 5, Figure 5.5, we show that if the machine learning prediction is lower than the threshold of the machine learning classifier (0.43), the result suggests that the English text is unlikely to be translated to difficult Japanese. The prior probability was based on the percentage of English texts that we translated to hard Japanese within the total English text database, and the likelihood ratios were based on a machine learning classifier's sensitivity and specificity (see https://www.cebm.ox.ac.uk/resources/ebm-tools/likelihood-ratios).

The right vertical illustrates both the positive posterior probability (the English will be translated as hard Japanese) and the negative posterior probability (the English text will be translated to easy Japanese). This result means that 1,000 in every 1,292 English texts with positive results, i.e., their estimated posterior probability larger than 0.43 will lead to Japanese translations which will have readability scores equal or smaller than 2.5.

This result also suggests that about 20 per cent of the predictions will be false positive, or English texts which will lead to readable Japanese translations but will be mis-classified as risky cases. This is however inevitable when selecting an optimal probability threshold of a machine learning classifier to increase both the sensitivity and cost-effectiveness of the model. To verify the accuracy of the predictive assessment, we compared two versions each of the Japanese translations of English texts. In each case the readability of the translation of the original English text was lower than that of the translation of the modified text. It was also found that the revision of the English texts resulted in translations which contained fewer characters of Chinese origin (Kango) and more of Japanese origin (Wago), the latter being generally considered as easier to read.

Chapter 6 addressed a persistent translation service challenge in multicultural countries whereby there is a shortage of properly qualified health translators proficient in African minority languages. For these languages, translation quality assurance presents a critical gap in multicultural health services. This chapter proposed to leverage machine learning techniques to devise a novel pre-editing approach. This approach would significantly boost the confidence of the developers of English environmental and health information for multicultural translation, engagement, promotion, and education. It would also help alleviate existing and increasing budgetary constraints on multicultural health service providers, through leveraging precise prediction of machine learning tools in improving the design and the translatability of English information. This chapter presented a continuation of the research approaches discussed in the previous chapter on Japanese translation readability prediction, to further illustrate the flexibility and adaptability of the proposed pre-editing strategy to improve the cost-effectiveness of quality control and assurance of environmental health translations in Asian and African languages.

This chapter looked at the situation in many countries where there is a shortage of health translators, and machine translation is seen as an option. The chapter presented a novel approach to predicting the accuracy of translations into four minority languages. Once again, corpus annotation of the English original texts was done using Readability Studio (lexicostatistical annotation). and USAS (semantic annotation). Machine Learning classification (to discriminate between texts likely to pick up errors in translation, and those likely to be translated perfectly) was done using Logistic Regression. Increasing the use of the percentage of proper nouns, percentage of unique words (type token ratio), and the percentage of words in the highest frequency category of the British National Corpus

(DiSp9), all reduced the rate of mistranslations into the African languages (as found by forward translation with Google followed by back translation with Bing). Texts are less translatable when increasing the use of less frequent and more formal words in the BNC (DiSp7), polysyllabic words or higher scores on the SMOG index. The percentage of numerals was not a statistically significant factor.

The final model selected was LR with seven features with z-score normalisation. We wanted to minimise the risk of false negatives, that is to say an English text classified as 'safe', but actually leading to mistranslations, so the probability threshold was set to its minimum value of 0.21. This meant that 75 per cent of the texts classified as safe were truly safe texts, while the other 25 per cent were false negatives. Five sample sentences were taken randomly from the set of sentences found to be 'risky' by the classifier. All had a predicted risk higher than 0.21 and thus were predicted to be 'risky' cases.

The second step was to revise the original English text to bring its risk probability score to below the threshold of 0.21. For example, one original English text ran 'The growth of the bacteria and the formation of toxins occur in products with low oxygen content and certain combinations of storage temperature and preservative parameters. This happens most often in lightly preserved foods and in inadequately processed, home canned or home-bottled foods.' The predicted probability of causing machine translation mistakes was 0.24, but by making changes such as increasing the number of unique words, the percentage of DiSp words, and reducing the number of multi-syllable and DiSp7 words, the revised form became 'Bacteria and other toxic content can grow in food kept at some temperatures or using certain ways to store them. This will not happen when food is stored properly with cans or bottles at home.' The probability of mistranslation of the revised text was reduced to 0.175. That the revision indeed was effective in reducing the risk of mistranslation was shown by both machine-translating the English texts (both original and revised) into each African language, and then translating back into English. Thus it was not necessary to know the African languages to see if errors had crept into the English texts during translation or back-translation. There were no errors in the back-translations of the revised English texts, but there were either two or three errors in the back-translations of the original English text. The advantage of this approach is that it is a cost-effective approach for increasing the confidence in machine translation of health-related texts to reach linguistic communities for whom there are not enough translators.

In Chapter 7, we looked at the readability of texts in Mandarin Chinese. A comparable corpus was built, to enable the comparison of texts produced by the China Centre of Disease Control (CCD), originally written in Chinese, and texts produced by the World Health Organization (WHO) which were translated into Chinese from other languages. Four different criteria were used to measure the readability of the texts: lexical difficulty (the ratio of difficult words to all words, where difficult words were defined as those not in the top 3,000 in a frequency list; semantic complexity (the number of polysemous words per sentence); orthographic complexity (the number of strokes per character) and information load defined by lexical density, the ratio of content words to all words. In each case the Mann Whitney U Test was used to show that the complexity of the CDC texts was significantly greater than that of the WHO texts. This finding tor the number of strokes per character was consistent with the study of the Dunn test in Chapter 2 where the number of strokes per character for WHO was found to be significantly less than that of either WHO or a third corpus produced by Merck's Manual of Diagnosis. The *Merck's Manual of Diagnosis* (MSD) data was collected from the MSD Website (Consumer Edition) Health topics https://www.msdmanuals.com/en-au/home.

Appendices

Appendix 4.1 Interpretation of the refined sixteen features

Original Annotation Tags	Interpretation
Number of unique three-syllable words	T=Types of multi-syllable words
A15	Abstract terms relating to (the level) of safety/danger
Wordy items	Verbose expressions
G1	Terms relating to government and governmental activities
Intrj_GI	Casual and slang words of dis/agreement
Nonadlt_GI	Words referring to infants through adolescents
Sv_GI	Verbs describing mental or emotional states
Affil_GI	Words of affiliation or supportiveness
Happiness_GALC	Words of happiness
Hostile_GI	Attitudes of hostility or aggressiveness
Vice_GI	Assessment of moral disapproval or misfortune
Number of complex three-syllable words	Tokens of multi-syllable words
Misspelling	Difficult words
You_GI	Second person pronouns
Fear_EmoLex	Emotions of fear, negative emotions
Compare_GI	Words of comparison

Appendix 5.1 Sources of English environmental health risk information

Bushfires and your health	https://www.healthdirect.gov.au/bushfires-and-your-health
Do face masks protect you from bushfire smoke?	https://www.healthdirect.gov.au/blog/do-face-masks-protect-you-from-bushfire-smoke
Burns and scalds	https://www.healthdirect.gov.au/burns-and-scalds
How to take medicines safely in a natural disaster (bushfire, floods, cyclones)	https://www.healthdirect.gov.au/blog/how-to-take-medicines-safely-in-a-natural-disaster
Natural disasters	https://www.healthdirect.gov.au/natural-disasters
What to do if you're feeling stressed or helpless about a natural disaster	https://www.healthdirect.gov.au/blog/what-to-do-if-youre-feeling-stressed-or-helpless-about-a-natural-disaster
Health risks after a cyclone or flood	https://www.healthdirect.gov.au/floods-and-cyclones
Dust storms	https://www.healthdirect.gov.au/dust-storms
Hot weather risks and staying cool	https://www.healthdirect.gov.au/hot-weather-risks-and-staying-cool
Sunburn and sun protection	https://www.healthdirect.gov.au/sunburn
Thunderstorm asthma	https://www.healthdirect.gov.au/thunderstorm-asthma
Leptospirosis	https://www.healthdirect.gov.au/leptospirosis
What's your plan? Before a flood	https://www.ses.nsw.gov.au/flood-awareness-nsw/
Do you live behind a levee?	https://www.ses.nsw.gov.au/floodsafe/learn-more-about-floods/do-you-live-behind-a-levee/
Floodsafe for rural areas	https://www.ses.nsw.gov.au/floodsafe/what-floodsafe-means-for-you/floodsafe-for-rural-areas/
Using sandbags to protect your home	https://www.ses.nsw.gov.au/floodsafe/prepare-your-home/during-a-flood/using-sandbags-to-protect-your-home/
The dangers of flash flooding	https://www.ses.nsw.gov.au/floodsafe/learn-more-about-floods/the-dangers-of-flash-flooding/
After flooding	https://www.ses.nsw.gov.au/floodsafe/prepare-your-home/after-flooding/
Next steps toward recovery	https://www.ses.nsw.gov.au/next-steps-toward-recovery/

(*cont.*)

Cleaning up after a flood	https://www.ses.nsw.gov.au/flood-resources/after-a-flood/cleaning-up-after-a-flood/
Know your risk	https://www.ses.nsw.gov.au/storm-resources/before-a-storm/know-your-risk/
Prepare your home	https://www.ses.nsw.gov.au/storm-resources/before-a-storm/prepare-your-home/
Look out for each other	https://www.ses.nsw.gov.au/storm-resources/during-a-storm/look-out-for-each-other/
Know your risk	https://www.ses.nsw.gov.au/storm-resources/after-a-storm/know-your-risk/
Volunteer	https://www.ses.nsw.gov.au/get-involved/volunteer/
Tsunami evacuation map	https://www.ses.nsw.gov.au/tsunamisafe/evacuation-map/tsunami-evacuation-map/
Know your risk	https://www.ses.nsw.gov.au/tsunami-resources/before-a-tsunami/know-your-risk/
Look out for each other	https://www.ses.nsw.gov.au/tsunami-resources/before-a-tsunami/look-out-for-each-other/
Bushfire overview	https://www.dfes.wa.gov.au/hazard-information/bushfire
Bushfires prepare	https://www.dfes.wa.gov.au/hazard-information/bushfire/prepare
During a bushfire	https://www.dfes.wa.gov.au/hazard-information/bushfire/during
Recovering from a bushfire	https://www.dfes.wa.gov.au/hazard-information/bushfire/recovery
Bushfire centre of excellence	https://www.dfes.wa.gov.au/hazard-information/bushfire/bcoe
Fires in the home	https://www.dfes.wa.gov.au/hazard-information/fire-in-the-home
Preventing a fire in the home	https://www.dfes.wa.gov.au/hazard-information/fire-in-the-home/preventing
Types of smoke alarms	https://www.dfes.wa.gov.au/hazard-information/fire-in-the-home/smoke-alarms
During a fire in the home	https://www.dfes.wa.gov.au/hazard-information/fire-in-the-home/during
Recovering from a fire in the home	https://www.dfes.wa.gov.au/hazard-information/fire-in-the-home/recovering
Cyclone Overview	https://www.dfes.wa.gov.au/hazard-information/cyclone
Prepare for a cyclone	https://www.dfes.wa.gov.au/hazard-information/cyclone/prepare#get-prepared

(*cont.*)

During a cyclone	https://www.dfes.wa.gov.au/hazard-information/cyclone/during
Recovering from a cyclone	https://www.dfes.wa.gov.au/hazard-information/cyclone/recovery
Storms overview	https://www.dfes.wa.gov.au/hazard-information/storm
Prepare for a storm	https://www.dfes.wa.gov.au/hazard-information/storm/prepare
During a storm	https://www.dfes.wa.gov.au/hazard-information/storm/during
Recovering from a storm	https://www.dfes.wa.gov.au/hazard-information/storm/recovery
Flood overview	https://www.dfes.wa.gov.au/hazard-information/flood
Prepare for a flood	https://www.dfes.wa.gov.au/hazard-information/flood/prepare
During a flood	https://www.dfes.wa.gov.au/hazard-information/flood/during
Recovering from a flood	https://www.dfes.wa.gov.au/hazard-information/flood/recovery
Flood risks under climate change	https://www.csiro.au/en/news/News-releases/2022/Flood-risks-under-climate-change
Northern Rivers Resilience Initiative	https://www.csiro.au/en/research/natural-disasters/floods/Northern-NSW-Resilience-Initiative
Understanding the causes and impacts of flooding	https://www.csiro.au/en/research/natural-disasters/floods/Causes-and-impacts
Tropical cyclones	https://www.csiro.au/en/research/natural-disasters/floods/FAQs-on-tropical-cyclones
Why don't our cities cope with heavy rain?	https://ecos.csiro.au/city-planning-for-heavy-rain/
Preparing Australia for future extreme bushfire events	https://www.csiro.au/en/research/natural-disasters/bushfires/Preparing-Australia
CSIRO Report on Climate and Disaster Resilience	https://www.csiro.au/en/research/natural-disasters/bushfires/report-climate-disaster-resilience
Understanding and managing bushfires	https://www.csiro.au/en/research/natural-disasters/bushfires/Understand-manage-bushfires
Predicting spotfire ignition in dry eucalypt litter	https://www.csiro.au/en/research/natural-disasters/bushfires/Spotfire-ignition
Bushfire assessment apps	https://www.csiro.au/en/research/natural-disasters/bushfires/Bushfire-Assessment
Smoke forecasting for bushfires and prescribed burns	https://www.csiro.au/en/research/natural-disasters/bushfires/Smoke-forecasting

(*cont.*)

Understanding loss of life in bushfires	https://www.csiro.au/en/research/natural-disasters/bushfires/Life-loss-database
Decadal climate forecasting	https://www.csiro.au/en/research/environmental-impacts/climate-change/Decadal-Forecasting
Atmospheric monitoring and modelling	https://www.csiro.au/en/research/natural-environment/atmosphere/Atmospheric-monitoring-modelling
NESP Earth Systems and Climate Change Hub	https://www.csiro.au/en/research/environmental-impacts/climate-change/ESCC-Hub
Oceans and climate change	https://www.csiro.au/en/research/natural-environment/oceans/Oceans-climate

Appendix 5.2 Examples of Japanese texts within different readability ranges

Lower-Elementary Text Example

I like music, so I often listen to CDs. I love Japan, so I study Japanese. I bought the CD because it was cheap. Disneyland was fun. The classroom was quiet. I like ramen noodles. I don't like cigarettes. Mr. Wang speaks good Japanese. I am not a good cook.

音楽がすきですから、よくCDを聞きます。日本がすきですから、日本語を勉強します。安かったですから、買いました。ディズニー ランドは楽しかったです。教室は静かでした。わたしはラー メンがすきです。わたしはたばこがきらいです。ワンさんは日本語が上手です。わたしは料理が下手です。

Upper-Elementary Text Example

Once upon a time, there was a king who loved gold. One day, an old man came to the king's house. The old man was a famous scholar, but he loved to drink. So the king prepared a lot of wine and delicious food for the old man. For ten days, the old man drank and ate. On the tenth day, he returned home satisfied. The god of wine heard this story. The god of wine liked the old man so much that he wanted to thank the king for his kindness.

むかしむかし、金が大好きな一 人の王様がいました。ある日王様の家に一 人の老人がやって来ました。その老人は有名な学者でしたが、お酒がたいへん好きでした。そこで、王様は、老人のためにたくさんの酒とおいしい料理を用意しました。 10 日間、老人は飲んだり食べたりしました。そして、10 日目に満足して帰って行きました。この話を、酒の神が聞きました。酒の神はこの老人が好きだったので、王様にお礼をしたいと思いました。

Lower-Intermediate Text Example

Once a week, the children gather at my grandmother's house with their grandchildren. It is very lively. For my grandmother's eightieth birthday, we rented the largest hotel in Manila and had over 500 people, including all members of her extended family and close friends. We feasted, danced, sang songs, and had a very lively time. My grandmother danced the waltz and the cha-cha-cha. Then all the children and grandchildren presented flowers.

毎週1回は祖母の家に子どもたちが孫たちをつれて集まります。とてもにぎやかです。祖母の 80 さいの誕生日には、マニラで一番大きなホテルを借りて、大家族の全員と親しい友人が、全部で 500 人以上集まりました。ごちそうを食べたり、ダンスをしたり、歌をうたったりして、とてもにぎやかでした。祖母もワルツやチャチャチャをおどりました。それから子どもと孫の全員が花をプレゼントしました。

Upper-Intermediate Text Example

What we now call renovation and recycling were taken as a matter of course. In Japan, the economy has been growing rapidly since the late 1950s, and the per capita income has been rising as the supply of goods increased rapidly. This period marked a reversal in the balance of supply and demand. Today, Japan is in a period of complete oversupply and under-demand. What do manufacturing companies do in such a situation?

いまでいうリフォーム、リサイクルをごく当たり前のこととしてやっていました。日本は、1950年代後半から経済の成長がいちじるしく、供給がどんどん増加し、国民一人あたりの所得も上がってきました。この時代を境にして、需要と供給のバランスが逆転しました。現在の日本は完全に供給が過剰、需要が不足している時代です。ものをつくる企業はこういうときにどうするでしょうか。

Lower-Advanced Text Example

The same is true for the movements of animals: rats scoot around a bit, and elephants move their feet slowly. Since ancient times, various people have investigated whether there is any relationship between body size and time. For example, they measured the time interval between heartbeats of mice, cats, dogs, horses, and elephants to determine the relationship between the weight of each animal and time. The reason for expressing size in terms of body weight is that body weight can be easily measured by simply placing it on a scale, but expressing size in terms of body length raises a number of difficult questions, such as whether the tail should be included in the measurement, and whether the length of the animal is measured when it is tall or when it is curled up.

動物の動きにしてもそうで、ネズミはちょこまかしているし、ゾウはゆっくりと足を運んでいく。体のサイズと時間との間に、何か関係があるのではないかと、古来、いろいろな人が調べてきた。例えば、心臓がドキン、ドキンと打つ時間間隔を、ネズミで測り、ネコで測り、イヌで測り、ウマで測り、ゾウで測り、と計測して、おのおのの動物の体重と時間との関係を求めてみたのである。サイズを体重で表わすのは、体重なら、はかりにポイと載せればすぐ測れるが、体長でサイズを表わすと、しっぽは計測値に入れるのか、背伸びした長さか丸まったときの長さかなどと、難しい問題がいろいろ出てくるからだ。

Upper-Advanced Text Example

Mathematics has the fundamental character of being a universal language for describing science. 'Nature is a book written in the language of mathematics', said Galilei. From Newton to the nineteenth century, classical physics and mathematics had developed in an inseparable relationship, with the study of differential equations and special functions as the 'linchpin' of the relationship. This development has led to a new era of mathematical physics. It has brought about new perspectives and tools that traverse not only analysis but also topology, varieties, algebraic geometry, and number theory, and has led to the solution of important problems and the development of new theories. Japan is home to many outstanding researchers in the field of mathematics, and their contributions to the development of this field around the world are worthy of special mention.

数学は，　科学を記述する普遍的な言語であるという基本的な性格を持つ。また「自然は数学の言葉で書かれた書物である」とはガリレイの言である。ニュートン以後19世紀まで，古典物理学と数学とは，微分方程式と特殊関数の研究を‘かなめ’として即かず離れずの関係で発展してきたが，今世紀に至り，場の量子論・統計力学と現代数学が結合し，　数理物理学の新しい発展を遂げることになった。この展開によって，　解析学のみでなくトポロジー，多様体論，代数幾何学，整数論にまでわたる，現代数学の先端諸分野を横断する新しい視点と手段がもたらされ，　重要な問題の解決や新しい理論の展開にまで導かれることになった。数学の分野において我が国は多数の優れた研究者を擁し，　世界のこの分野の発展に大きく貢献した業績は特筆すべきものがある。

Appendix 6.1 Sources of English environmental health information

Alcohol	https://www.who.int/news-room/fact-sheets/detail/alcohol
Ambient (outdoor) air pollution	https://www.who.int/news-room/fact-sheets/detail/ambient-(outdoor)-air-quality-and-health
Animal bites	https://www.who.int/news-room/fact-sheets/detail/animal-bites
Arsenic	https://www.who.int/news-room/fact-sheets/detail/arsenic
Asbestos: elimination of asbestos-related diseases	https://www.who.int/news-room/fact-sheets/detail/asbestos-elimination-of-asbestos-related-diseases
Asthma	https://www.who.int/news-room/fact-sheets/detail/asthma
Biodiversity and health	https://www.who.int/news-room/fact-sheets/detail/biodiversity-and-health
Blood safety and availability	https://www.who.int/news-room/fact-sheets/detail/blood-safety-and-availability
Botulism	https://www.who.int/news-room/fact-sheets/detail/botulism
Brucellosis	https://www.who.int/news-room/fact-sheets/detail/brucellosis
Burns	https://www.who.int/news-room/fact-sheets/detail/burns
Buruli ulcer (Mycobacterium ulcerans infection)	https://www.who.int/news-room/fact-sheets/detail/buruli-ulcer-(mycobacterium-ulcerans-infection)

(*cont.*)

Chagas disease (also known as American trypanosomiasis)	https://www.who.int/news-room/fact-sheets/detail/chagas-disease-(american-trypanosomiasis)
Child mortality (under 5 years)	https://www.who.int/news-room/fact-sheets/detail/levels-and-trends-in-child-under-5-mortality-in-2020
Cholera	https://www.who.int/news-room/fact-sheets/detail/cholera
Chronic obstructive pulmonary disease (COPD)	https://www.who.int/news-room/fact-sheets/detail/chronic-obstructive-pulmonary-disease-(copd)
Climate change and health	https://www.who.int/news-room/fact-sheets/detail/climate-change-and-health
Crimean-Congo haemorrhagic fever	https://www.who.int/news-room/fact-sheets/detail/crimean-congo-haemorrhagic-fever
Deafness and hearing loss	https://www.who.int/news-room/fact-sheets/detail/deafness-and-hearing-loss
Dengue and severe dengue	https://www.who.int/news-room/fact-sheets/detail/dengue-and-severe-dengue
Dioxins and their effects on human health	https://www.who.int/news-room/fact-sheets/detail/dioxins-and-their-effects-on-human-health
Dracunculiasis (guinea-worm disease)	https://www.who.int/news-room/fact-sheets/detail/dracunculiasis-(guinea-worm-disease)
Drinking-water	https://www.who.int/news-room/fact-sheets/detail/drinking-water
Drowning	https://www.who.int/news-room/fact-sheets/detail/drowning
Looking after your health in lockdown	https://cid.org.au/wp-content/uploads/2021/08/Looking-after-your-health-in-lock down.pdf
Supporting people in group homes with a COVID outbreak	https://cid.org.au/wp-content/uploads/2021/07/Plain-English-Guide-about-Supporting-people-in-group-homes.pdf
What is happening in my home	https://cid.org.au/resource/what-is-happening-in-my-home/
Wearing masks during Coronavirus	https://cid.org.au/wp-content/uploads/2020/08/Wearing-masks-during-Coronavirus-Info-guide-CID.pdf
My safety plan	https://cid.org.au/wp-content/uploads/2020/07/My-Safety-Plan-CID-Jul20.pdf
COVID-19 Leave no one behind	https://cid.org.au/wp-content/uploads/2020/07/COVID-19-Leave-no-one-behind-Easy-Read-CID-Jun20.pdf

(*cont.*)

If you think you have Coronavirus	https://cid.org.au/wp-content/uploads/2020/08/If-you-think-you-have-Coronavirus-info-guide-CID.pdf
Looking after your health during Coronavirus	https://cid.org.au/wp-content/uploads/2020/08/Looking-after-your-health-during-Coronavirus-Easy-Read-CID.pdf
Staying safe from house fires	https://cid.org.au/wp-content/uploads/2020/06/Staying-safe-from-house-fires-CID-Jun20.pdf
Viruses and staying healthy	https://cid.org.au/wp-content/uploads/2020/03/Viruses-staying-healthy-Council-Intellectual-Disability.pdf
How to cope in a heatwave	https://cid.org.au/wp-content/uploads/2019/12/How-to-cope-in-a-heatwave-Council-intellectual-disability.pdf
Mental health	https://cid.org.au/wp-content/uploads/2019/12/HFS-ER-Mental-health.pdf
Tips to help mental health	https://cid.org.au/wp-content/uploads/2019/07/Tips-to-help-mental-health.pdf
Me and my doctor	https://cid.org.au/wp-content/uploads/2019/11/Me-and-my-doctor-health-guide.pdf
After visiting the doctor	https://cid.org.au/wp-content/uploads/2019/11/After-visiting-the-doctor-health-guide.pdf
Finding a new doctor	https://cid.org.au/wp-content/uploads/2019/11/Finding-a-new-doctor-health-guide.pdf
Me and my medication	https://cid.org.au/wp-content/uploads/2019/11/Me-and-my-medication-health-guide.pdf
Wellbeing is important	https://cid.org.au/wp-content/uploads/2023/03/ER-Wellbeing.pdf
COVID-19 medicines	https://cid.org.au/wp-content/uploads/2022/08/covid-19-medicines-easy-read.pdf
Health Position Statement 2022	https://cid.org.au/wp-content/uploads/2022/08/Health_position_statement_Easy_Read_2022.pdf
Info about the flu vaccine	https://cid.org.au/wp-content/uploads/2022/07/information-about-the-flu-vaccine-easy-read-information-about-the-flu-vaccine.pdf
Top issues for people with intellectual disability this election	https://cid.org.au/wp-content/uploads/2022/05/ER-Election-Asks-May-2022.pdf
What to do if you get COVID	https://cid.org.au/wp-content/uploads/2022/02/Health-ER-COVID-19-Guide-print.pdf
Booster doses of the COVID vaccine fact sheet	https://cid.org.au/resource/booster-doses-of-the-covid-vaccine/

(*cont.*)

The third dose of the COVID vaccine fact sheet	https://cid.org.au/wp-content/uploads/2021/12/Health-ER-Fact-sheet-3rd-dose-Covid-vaccine-digital-accessible.pdf
Here's how we do advocacy at CID	https://cid.org.au/wp-content/uploads/2021/07/Advocating-for-Our-Health-Counts.pdf
Yearly health checks	https://cid.org.au/wp-content/uploads/2021/09/Yearly-Health-Check-Easy-Read-Fact-Sheet.pdf
Your right to good health care	https://cid.org.au/wp-content/uploads/2021/09/Your-right-to-good-health-care-Easy-Read-Fact-Sheet.pdf
Types of health checks	https://cid.org.au/wp-content/uploads/2021/09/Types-of-Health-Checks-Easy-Read-Fact-Sheet.pdf
Caring for your teeth fact sheet	https://cid.org.au/wp-content/uploads/2021/09/Caring-for-your-teeth-Easy-Read-Fact-Sheet.pdf
Chronic health plans fact sheet	https://cid.org.au/wp-content/uploads/2021/09/Chronic-Health-Plans-Easy-Read-Fact-Sheet.pdf
Adult health services	https://cid.org.au/wp-content/uploads/2021/09/Adult-Health-Services-Easy-Read-Fact-Sheet.pdf
Abdominal aortic aneurysm	https://www.nhsinform.scot/illnesses-and-conditions/heart-and-blood-vessels/conditions/abdominal-aortic-aneurysm/
Acute cholecystitis	https://www.nhsinform.scot/illnesses-and-conditions/stomach-liver-and-gastrointestinal-tract/acute-cholecystitis/
Allergic rhinitis	https://www.nhsinform.scot/illnesses-and-conditions/ears-nose-and-throat/allergic-rhinitis/
Anal cancer	https://www.nhsinform.scot/illnesses-and-conditions/cancer/cancer-types-in-adults/anal-cancer/
Asthma	https://www.nhsinform.scot/illnesses-and-conditions/lungs-and-airways/asthma/
Bipolar disorder	https://www.nhsinform.scot/illnesses-and-conditions/mental-health/bipolar-disorder/
Bone cancer	https://www.nhsinform.scot/illnesses-and-conditions/cancer/cancer-types-in-adults/bone-cancer/
Brain stem death	https://www.nhsinform.scot/illnesses-and-conditions/brain-nerves-and-spinal-cord/brain-stem-death/

(*cont.*)

Cold sore	https://www.nhsinform.scot/illnesses-and-conditions/mouth/cold-sore/
Coma	https://www.nhsinform.scot/illnesses-and-conditions/brain-nerves-and-spinal-cord/coma/
Common cold	https://www.nhsinform.scot/illnesses-and-conditions/infections-and-poisoning/common-cold/
Cough	https://www.nhsinform.scot/illnesses-and-conditions/lungs-and-airways/cough/
Croup	https://www.nhsinform.scot/illnesses-and-conditions/lungs-and-airways/croup/#about-croup
Alcohol and the immune system	https://www.ncbi.nlm.nih.gov/pmc/articles/PMC4590612/
Alcohol and gut-derived inflammation	https://www.ncbi.nlm.nih.gov/pmc/articles/PMC5513683/
The respiratory risks of ambient/outdoor air pollution	https://www.ncbi.nlm.nih.gov/pmc/articles/PMC7665094/
Animal bites	https://www.ncbi.nlm.nih.gov/books/NBK430852/
Arsenic in rice: Should you be concerned?	https://www.healthline.com/nutrition/arsenic-in-rice
Asthma	https://www.ncbi.nlm.nih.gov/books/NBK430901/
Biodiversity, drug discovery, and the future of global health: Introducing the biodiversity to biomedicine consortium, a call to action	https://www.ncbi.nlm.nih.gov/pmc/articles/PMC5735771/
Coronavirus disease 2019: Coronaviruses and blood safety	https://www.ncbi.nlm.nih.gov/pmc/articles/PMC7135848/

Appendix 7.1 Sources of Chinese health information – Original Chinese

Infectious Disease Control and Prevention Institute
Viral Disease Control and Prevention Institute
Parasitic Disease Prevention and Control Centre
STD and AIDS Prevention and Control Centre
Chronic Non-communicable Disease Prevention and Control Centre
Nutrition and Health Institute Environment and Health-Related Product Safety Institute

Institute of Occupational Health and Poison Control Radiation Protection and Nuclear Safety Medicine
Rural Water Improvement Technology Guidance Centre
Maternal and Child Health Centre
China Association for STD and AIDS Prevention and Control
Chinese Nutrition Society
China Hepatitis Prevention Foundation
Preventive Medicine Information Committee of Chinese Preventive Medicine Association

Appendix 7.2 Examples of Chinese polysemous words

安	safe, secure, quiet, calm, content, satisfied, still, install, fit, pacify, fix
熬	boil, decoct, endure, hard to bear, survive, stuck, stay up, suffer, torture
把握	grasp, seize, take advantage of, hold, certainty, assurance, sure, control, confidence
搬	move, carry, back, relocate, copy indiscriminately, shift, freight, removal
拨	dial, call, allocate, redial, pluck, push aside, provoke, devote, set right
布置	arrange, furnish, decorate, assign, appoint, posit, layout, setup, deploy, put in order
裁	cut, trim, reduce, diminish, cut back, downsize, decide, abolish, judge, redundancy
藏	hide, stash, conceal, harbor, treasure, secret, store, contain, collect, Tibet
操纵	manipulate, control, rig, operate, steer, handle, fix, drive, navigate, manoeuvre
插	insert, stick in, pierce, take part in, interfere, interpose, plug-in, illustration, jump a queue
拆	open up, tear down, demolish, dismantle, remove, destroy, expose, separate, take apart
搀	take by the arm and assist, mix, blend, dilute, involve, interfere, mingle, debase, meddle
缠	wind around, wrap round, entangle, coil, tangle, involve, bother, annoy, knot, twine
抄	copy, plagiarise, cheat, search, seize, raid, grab, take a shortcut, extract, handwritten
超过	surpass, exceed, outstrip, beyond, overstep, more than, over, above, overtake, outweigh
吵	quarrel, fight, make a noise, noisy, disturb, annoying, loud, bother, racket, clamour, uproar
撤	remove, take away, withdraw, recall, dismiss, replace, leave, pull out, retreat, evacuate
闯	rush, break, intrude, crash through a barrier, adventure, well-travelled, get into trouble, failing to stop
称	call, say, to name, claim, term, argue, describe, to weigh, praise, suitable, well qualified
成立	set up, establish, form, create, launch, tenable, reasonable, found, completion

(*cont.*)

承认	admit, concede, recognise, acknowledge, plea, confess, accept, approval
乘	ride, mount, catch, multiply, follow up, take advantage of, seize the opportunity
除	get rid of, delete, remove, exclude, eliminate, divide, except, not including, unless
答应	promise, agree, permit, reply, answer, respond, accept, consent, offer, comply, deal
代表	representative, delegate, represent, stand for, on behalf of, in the name of, mean, indicate

Appendix 7.3 Examples of lexical density in Chinese health information for the public

Technical terms (TT), Proper nouns (PN), Names of diseases and chemicals (NA)

Air Pollution – Source: WHO

空气污染 指 任何 改变大气 **自然特征 (TT)** 的化学, 物理或生物因素对室内或室外环境的污染。
Air pollution is the contamination of the indoor or outdoor environment by any chemical, physical, or biological factor that alters the **natural characteristics of the atmosphere** (TT).

从 城市 上空 的 雾霾 到 室内 的 烟雾, 空气污染 构成了 重大 健康威胁 和 气候威胁。
From the haze that hangs over cities to the smoke indoors, air pollution poses a major health and climate threat.

城市和农村地区的 环境 (室外) 空气污染 正在 产生 **细颗粒物 (NA)**, 导致 **中风 (NA), 心脏病 (NA), 肺癌 (NA)**, 急性和 **慢性呼吸道疾病 (NA)**。
Ambient (outdoor) air pollution in urban and rural areas is producing **fine particulate matter (NA)** that causes stroke (NA), **heart disease** (NA), **lung cancer** (NA), and acute and **chronic respiratory diseases** (NA).

此外, 约有26亿人因使用以煤油, 生物质 (木柴、动物粪便、作物废弃物) 和煤炭为燃料的污染性 明火 或 简陋 炉灶 进行 烹饪 而 暴露在 **危险水平 (TT)** 的家庭空气污染中。
In addition, about 2.6 billion people are exposed to **hazardous levels (TT)** of household air pollution from cooking on polluting open fires or crude

cookers fuelled by paraffin, biomass (firewood, animal dung, crop waste) and coal.

环境 空气污染 和 家庭空气污染 的 综合影响 每年 导致 约700万人过早死亡。
The combined effects of ambient air pollution and household air pollution cause about seven million premature deaths each year.

空气污染的来源是多方面的，并且因环境而异。主要的 室外污染源 包括 用于 烹饪 和 取暖 的 住宅能源、车辆、发电、 农业/废弃物 焚烧 和 工业。支持 可持续 土地利用、更清洁 的 家庭能源和交通、节能住宅、发电、工业和更好的城市垃圾管理的政策和投资，可以有效减少环境空气污染的主要来源。
Sources of air pollution are multiple and vary from one environment to another. Major outdoor sources include residential energy for cooking and heating, vehicles, electricity generation, agriculture/waste incineration and industry. Policies and investments that support sustainable land use, cleaner household energy and transport, energy-efficient homes, electricity generation, industry and better municipal waste management can be effective in reducing major sources of ambient air pollution.

Air Pollution – CCDC

污染天气是指在无风、**逆温** (TT) 和高湿等不利气象条件下，污染物在空气中堆积导致的空气污染现象。重污染天气一般是指 **空气质量指数** (TT) 大于200，即 **环境空气质量** (TT) 达到 重度及以上 污染程度的 空气污染现象。
Polluted weather is an air pollution phenomenon caused by the accumulation of pollutants in the air under unfavourable meteorological conditions such as windlessness, temperature inversion (TT) and high humidity. Heavily polluted weather is generally defined as an air pollution phenomenon where the Air Quality Index (TT) is greater than 200, i.e., the ambient air quality (TT) reaches a level of heavy pollution or above.

以**PM2.5 (TT)**为 首要污染物 的 重污染天气 俗称 '雾霾'。可能发生重污染天气时，地方政府将发布 预警信息。
Heavily polluted weather with PM2.5 (TT) as the main pollutant is commonly known as 'haze'. Local governments issue warnings when heavy polluted weather is likely to occur.

大气中的 **PM2.5 (TT)** 为 **直径 (TT)**小于或等于2.5 **微米** (TT) 的所有**颗粒物** (TT) 的总称, 其 直径 约为 头发丝的二十分之一。PM2.5在大气中可以停留较长时间, 不容易去除, 且能吸附多种有害物质, 容易被吸入呼吸道深部, 某些组分还可进入血液, 危害人体健康。
PM2.5 (TT) in the atmosphere is a general term for all particulate matter (TT) with a diameter (TT) less than or equal to 2.5 microns (TT), whose diameter is about one twentieth that of a hairline. PM2.5 can stay in the atmosphere for a long time, is not easy to remove, and can adsorb a variety of hazardous substances, which can be easily inhaled into the deep respiratory tract, and some components can enter the bloodstream, endangering human health.

以**PM2.5 (TT)** 为首要污染物的重污染天气的急性危害主要表现为短时间内吸入污染物引起的咳嗽、咽喉痛、眼部刺激等症状。重污染天气还可诱发 **支气管哮喘 (NA)**、**慢性阻塞性肺疾病 (NA)**、**心脑血管疾病 (NA)** 等 **慢性疾病** (NA) 的急性发作 或 病情加重。
The acute hazards of heavy polluted weather, with PM2.5 (TT) as the main pollutant, are mainly symptoms such as cough, sore throat and eye irritation caused by inhaling pollutants for a short period of time. Heavy pollution can also trigger acute attacks or aggravation of chronic diseases (NA) such as bronchial asthma (NA), chronic obstructive pulmonary disease (COPD), and cardiovascular disease (NA).

选购 空气净化器时, 要注意选择符合 国家标准 的 空气净化器 (GB/T 18801–2015《空气净化器》), 主要 参考 两类 **指标 (TT)**, 即 **洁净空气量** (TT) 和 **累积净化量 (TT)**。
When choosing an air purifier, it is important to select an air purifier that complies with the national standard (GB/T 18801–2015 'Air Purifier'), with reference to two types of indicators (TT), i.e., Clean Air Volume (TT) and Cumulative Purification Volume (TT).

净化器 的 **适用面积** (TT) 可以 **用** **颗粒物CADR值 (TT)** 乘以0.1来估算 (比如, **颗粒物CADR (TT)** 为300 m3/h的 空气净化器, 适用面积约为30 m2) 。**CCM值 (TT)** 反映了 净化部件 的 使用寿命 (**CCM数值 (TT)** 越大, 净化部件的更换或清洗周期越长) 。
The applicable area (TT) of the purifier can be estimated by multiplying the particulate CADR (TT) by 0.1 (e.g., an air purifier with a particulate CADR (TT) of 300 m3/h would have an applicable area of about 30 m2), and the CCM value (TT) reflects the lifespan of the purification components (the higher the CCM value (TT), the longer the cycle of replacing or cleaning of purification components).

Appendix 7.4 Paired-sample area difference under the receiver operating characteristic curves

	Asymptotic				Asymptotic 95% Confidence Interval	
Test Result Pair(s)	z	Sig. (2-tail)[a]	AUC Difference	Std. Error Difference[b]	Lower Bound	Upper Bound
Density of content words vs. Index	−1.521	0.128	−0.044	0.214	−0.100	0.013
Density of content words vs. Ratio of Difficult Words	−0.690	0.490	−0.019	0.215	−0.073	0.035
Density of content words vs. Average Strokes per character	1.107	0.268	0.036	0.219	−0.028	0.099
Density of content words vs. Ratio of sentences with complex semantic categories	0.665	0.506	0.022	0.220	−0.043	0.088
Index vs. Ratio of Difficult Words	1.327	0.184	0.025	0.209	−0.012	0.062
Index vs. Average Strokes per character	6.378	0.000 **	0.080	0.212	0.055	0.104
Index vs. Ratio of sentences with complex semantic categories	2.357	0.018 **	0.066	0.214	0.011	0.121

(*cont.*)

Test Result Pair(s)	Asymptotic z	Asymptotic Sig. (2-tail)[a]	AUC Difference	Std. Error Difference[b]	Asymptotic 95% Confidence Interval Lower Bound	Asymptotic 95% Confidence Interval Upper Bound
Ratio of Difficult Words vs. Average Strokes per character	2.326	0.020 **	0.055	0.214	0.009	0.101
Ratio of Difficult Words vs. Ratio of sentences with complex semantic categories	1.272	0.203	0.041	0.216	−0.022	0.105
Average Strokes per character vs. Ratio of sentences with complex semantic categories	-0.373	0.709	−0.014	0.220	−0.085	0.058

a. Null hypothesis: true area difference = 0

b. Under the nonparametric assumption

References

Agarwal, N., Hansberry, D.R., Sabourin, V., Tomei, K.L., & Prestigiacomo, C.J. (2013). A comparative analysis of the quality of patient education materials from medical specialties. *JAMA Internal Medicine* 173(13), 1257.

Akhlaq, A., McKinstry, B., Muhammad, K.B., & Sheikh, A. (2016). Barriers and facilitators to health information exchange in low- and middle-income country settings: A systematic review. *Health Policy and Planning* 31(9), 1310–1325.

Altman, D.G. (1991). *Practical statistics for medical research*. Boca Raton, FL: Chapman and Hall / CRC Press.

Aluisi, S., Specia, L., Gasperin, C., & Scarton, C. Readability assessment for text simplification. *Proc NAACL HLT 2021 fifth workshop on innovative use of NLP for building educational applications* (pp. 1–9).

Azpiazu, I.M., & Pera, M.S. (2019). Multiattentive recurrent neural network architecture for multilingual readability assessment. *Transactions of the Association for Computational Linguistics* 7, 421–436.

Azpiazu, I.M. & Pera, M.S. (2020). Is cross-lingual readability assessment possible? *Journal of the Association for Information Science and Technology* 71(6), 644–456.

Baayen, R.H. (2008). *Analyzing linguistic data: A practical introduction to statistics using R*. Cambridge: Cambridge University Press.

Bailin, A., & Grafstein, A. (2001). The linguistic assumptions underlying readability formulae. *Language & Communication* 21(3), 285–301.

Balakrishnan, V., Chandy, Z., Hseih, A., Bui, T.L., & Verma, S.P. (2016). Readability and understandability of online vocal cord paralysis materials. *Otolaryngology–Head and Neck Surgery* 154(3), 460–464.

Basch, C.H., Mohlman, J., Hillyer, G.C., & Garcia, P. (2020). Public health communication in time of crisis: Readability of on-line COVID-19 information. *Disaster Medicine and Public Health Preparedness* 14(5), 635–637.

Beaunoyer, E., Arsenault, M., Lomanowska, A.M., & Guitton, M.J. (2017). Understanding online health information: Evaluation, tools, and strategies. *Patient Education and Counseling* 100(2), 183–189.

Benoit, J-P. (1986). Revue critique de formules de lisibilité (60 ans de formules de lisibilité: qu'en reste-t-il?). *Pratiques de lecture* 52, 45–63.

Berland, G.K., Elliott, M.N., Morales, L.S., Algazy, J.I., Kravitz, R.L., Broder, M. S., et al. (2001). Health information on the internet. *JAMA* 285(20), 2612.

Björnsson, C.H. (1968). *Läsbarhet.* Stockholm: Liber.

Boholm, M., Möller, N., & Hansson, S.O. (2015). The concepts of risk, safety, and security: Applications in everyday language. *Risk Analysis* 36(2), 320–338.

Braga-Neto, U.M., & Dougherty, E.R. (2004). Is cross-validation valid for small-sample microarray classification? *Bioinformatics* 20(3), 374–380.

Buller, D.B., Burgoon, M., Hall, J.R., Levine, N., Taylor, A.M., Beach, B.H., et al. (2000). Using language intensity to increase the success of a family intervention to protect children from ultraviolet radiation: Predictions from language expectancy theory. *Preventive Medicine* 30(2), 103–113.

Buse, R.P.L, & Westley, R.W. (2008). A metric for software readability (pp. 121–130). ISTTA, 20–24 July, Seattle, Washington, USA.

Butler, C. (1985). *Statistics in linguistics.* New York: Basil Blackwell.

Carter, I. (1999). Serial No. 31: Locally generated printed materials in agriculture: Experience from Uganda and Ghana. Department for International Development Education Research Report. London: Department for International Development.

Carter, I. (2005). Creating locally relevant health information. *PLoS Medicine* 2(3), e46. https://doi.org/10.1371/journal.pmed.0020046

Carter, R., Adolphs, S., Brown, B., Crawford, P., & Sahota, O. (2007). Applying corpus linguistics in a health care context. *Journal of Applied Linguistics* 1(1), 9–28.

Caylor, J.S., Sticht, T.G., Fox, L.C., & Ford, J.P. (1972). Methodologies for determining reading requirements for military occupational specialities. *Human Resources Research Organization*, Technical Report.

Charnock, D., Shepperd, S., Needham, G., & Gann, R. (1999). DISCERN: An instrument for judging the quality of written consumer health information on treatment choices. *Journal of Epidemiology & Community Health* 53(2), 105–111.

Chinese Knowledge Information Processing (CKIP). (1993). Chinese Electronic Dictionary. Technical Report, No. 93–05. Taiwan: Academia Sinica.

Cohen, M.S., Henderson, G.E., Aiello, P., & Zheng, H. (1996). Successful eradication of sexually transmitted diseases in the People's Republic of China: Implications for the 21st century. *Journal of Infectious Dis*eases 174(Suppl. 2), S223–229.

Coleman, M., & Liau, T.L. (1975). A computer readability formula designed for machine scoring. *Journal of Applied Psychology* 60, 283–284.

Collins-Thompson, K., & Callan, J. (2004). A language modelling approach to predicting reading difficulty. *Proc HLT/NAACL* (pp. 100–193).

Correia, J., & Mendes, R. (2021). Neural complexity assessment: A deep learning approach to readability classification for European Portuguese corpora. Intelligent Data Engineering and Automated Learning (IDEAL) 22nd International Conference, Manchester, UK, 25–27 November.

Council of Europe (CoE). (2001). *Common European Framework of Reference for Languages: Learning, teaching, assessment.* Cambridge: Cambridge University Press.

Covello, V. T. (1992). Risk communication: An emerging area of health communication research. *Annals of the International Communication Association* 15(1), 359–373.

Crawford, P., Brown, B., & Harvey, K. (2014). Corpus linguistics and evidence-based health communication. In Heidi Hamilton, Wen-ying Sylvia Chou (eds.), *The Routledge handbook of language and health communication* (Routledge Handbooks in Applied Linguistics). London: Routledge.

Cronin, M. (2003). *Translation and globalization*. London: Routledge.

Crossley, S., Allan, D.B., & McNamara, D.S. (2011). Text readability and intuitive simplification : A comparison of readability formula. *Reading in a Foreign Language* 23(1), 84–101.

Crossley, S.A., Balyan, R., Liu, J., Karter, A.J., McNamara, D., & Schillinger, D. (2020). Predicting the readability of physicians' secure messages to improve health communication using novel linguistic features: Findings from the ECLIPPSE study. *Journal of Communication in Healthcare* 13(4), 344–356.

Crossley, S.A., Kyle, K., & McNamara, D.S. (2016). Sentiment Analysis and Social Cognition Engine (SEANCE): An automatic tool for sentiment, social cognition, and social-order analysis. *Behavior Research Methods* 49(3), 803–821.

Crystal, A., & Greenberg, J. (2006). Relevance criteria identified by health information users during Web searches. *Journal of the American Society for Information Science and Technology* 57(10), 1368–1382.

Curtotti, M., McCreath, E., Bruce, T., Frug, S., Weibel, W., & Ceynowa, N. (2015). Machine learning for readability of legislative sentences. ICAIL, 8–12, June, San Diego, CA, USA.

D'Alessandro, D.M., Kingsley, P., & Johnson-West, J. (2001). The readability of pediatric patient education materials on the world wide web. *Archives of Pediatrics & Adolescent Medicine* 155(7), 807.

Dale, E., & Chall, J.S. (1949). The concept of readability. *Elementary English* 26(23), 19–26.

Dale, E., & Tyler, R.W. (1934). A study of the factors influencing the difficulty of reading materials for adults of limited reading ability. *Library Quarterly* 4, 384–412.

De Mauro, T. (2000). Il dizionario della lingua italiana. Torino: Paravia.

Deutsch, T., Jasbi, M., & Shieber, S. (2020). Linguistic features for readability assessment. In *Proceedings of the 15th Workshop on Innovative use of NLP for Building Educational Applications* (pp. 1–17), 10 July.

Diederich, J., Kindermann, J., Leopold, E., & Paass, G. (2003). Authorship attribution with support vector machines. *Applied Intelligence* 19, 109–123.

Doherty, M., Beusenberg, M., Asamoah-Odei, E., Lule, F., Pendse, R., Ghidinelli, M., et al. (2015). Rapid uptake and adoption of the WHO 2013 consolidated ARV guidelines recommendations: Paving the way to achieving 90/90/90 global target. *Journal of the International AIDS Society* 18. https://doi.org/10.7448/IAS.18.5.20345

Doubleday, A.R., Novin, S., Long, K.L., Schneider, D.F., Sippel, R.S, & Pitt, S. C. (2021). Online information for treatment for low-risk thyroid cancer: Assessment of timeliness, content, quality, and readability. *Journal of Cancer Education* 36, 850–857.

du Toit, E. (2017). The readability of integrated reports. *Meditari Accountancy Research* 25(4), 629–653.

Eastin, M.S. (2006). Credibility assessments of online health information: The effects of source expertise and knowledge of content. *Journal of Computer-Mediated Communication* 6(4), JCMC643. https://doi.org/10.1111/j.1083-6101.2001.tb00126.x

Elder, J.P., Ayala, G.X., Parra-Medina, D., & Talavera, G.A. (2009). Health communication in the Latino community: Issues and approaches. *Annual Review of Public Health* 30(1), 227–251.

Ennis, M., McKay, B., Mylan, L., Dyke, E., & Deonandan, R. (2016). Evaluation of the impact of WHO publications. Corporate evaluation commissioned by the WHO Evaluation Office, Ontario, Canada. Available at: https://www.who.int/docs/default-source/documents/evaluation/report-evaluation-impact-who-publications.pdf?sfvrsn=577627c5_2

Falkenjack, J., Heimann Mühlenbock, K., Jönsson, A. Features indicating readability in Swedish text. *Proceedings of the 10th Nordic Conference of Computational Linguistics* (NODALIDA 2013): *Linköping Electronic Conference Proceedings* 85, 27.

Feng, L., Jansche M., & Huenerfauth, N. (2010). A comparison of features for automatic readability assessment. *Proceedings of the 12th Conference of the European Chapter of the Association for Computational Linguistics*, pp. 229–237.

Field, A. (2000). *Discovering statistics using IBM SPSS statistics*. Fourth Edition. Los Angeles, CA: Sage Publications.

Flesch, R. (1948). A new readability yardstick. *Journal of Applied Psychology* 32(3), 221–223.

Flesch, R. (1950). Measuring the level of abstraction. *Journal of Applied Psychology* 34(6), 384–390.

Flesch, R. (1952). 'Simplification of Flesch Reading Ease Formula': Reply. *Journal of Applied Psychology* 36(1), 54–55.

Francina, V., & Vacca, R. (1986). Adaptation of Flesch readability index on a bilingual text written by the same author both in Italian and English languages. *Linguaggi* 3, 47–49.

François, T., & Fairon, C. (2012). An 'AI readability' formula for French as a foreign language. *Proceedings of the 2001 Joint Conference on Empirical Methods in Natural Language Processing and Computational Natural Language Learning* (pp. 466–477), Jeju Island, Korea, 12–14 July.

Friedman, D.B., & Hoffman-Goetz, L. (2006). A systematic review of readability and comprehension instruments used for print and web-based cancer information. *Health Education & Behavior* 33(3), 352–373.

Fritz, C.O., Morris, P.E., & Richler, J.J. (2012). Effect size estimates: Current use, calculations, and interpretation. *Journal of Experimental Psychology: General* 141(1), 2–18.

Fry, E.B. (1968). A readability formula that saves time. *Journal of Reading* 11, 513–516.

Garner, S. (1995). WEKA: The Waikato Environment for Knowledge Analysis. *Proceedings of the New Zealand Computer Science Research Students' Conference*, May.

Golding, D., Krimsky, S., & Plough, A. (1992). Evaluating risk communication: Narrative vs. technical presentations of information about radon. *Risk Analysis* 12(1), 27–35. https://doi.org/10.1111/j.1539-6924.1992.tb01304.x

Gowan, M.E., Sloan, J.A., & Kirk, R.C. (2015). Prepared for what? Addressing the disaster readiness gap beyond preparedness for survival. *BMC Public Health* 15(1), 1–5.

Gray, W.S., & Leary, B.E. (1935). *What makes a book readable.* Chicago, IL: University of Chicago Press.

Gray, N.J., Klein, J.D., Noyce, P.R., Sesselberg, T.S., & Cantrill, J.A. (2005). Health information-seeking behaviour in adolescence: The place of the internet. *Social Science & Medicine* 60(7), 1467–1478.

Gunning, R. (1952). *The technique of clear writing* (pp. 36–37). New York: McGraw-Hill.

Gunning, R. (1969). The Fog Index after twenty years. *Journal of Business Communication* 6(2), 3–13.

Haberlandt, K.F., & Graesser, A.C. (1985). Component processes in text comprehension and some of their interactions. *Journal of Experimental Psychology: General, 114*(3), 357–374. https://doi.org/10.1037/0096-3445.114.3.357

Hagemeier-Klose, M., & Wagner, K. (2009). Evaluation of flood hazard maps in print and web mapping services as information tools in flood risk communication. *Natural Hazards and Earth System Sciences* 9(2), 563–574.

Han, C.X. (2019). Statistics in corpus linguistics: A practical guide *Journal of Quantitative Linguistics* 27(4), 379–383. https://doi.org/10.1080/09296174.2019.1646069

Hansberry, D., Agarwal, N., Gonzales, S., & Baker, S. (2014). Are we effectively informing patients? A quantitative analysis of on-line patient education resources from the American Society of Neuroradiology. *American Journal of Neuroradiology* 35(7), 1270–1275.

Harvey, K., & Koteyko, N. (2013). *Exploring health communication.* London: Routledge.

Harvey, K., Mahlberg, M., & Teubert, W. (2015). Investigating adolescent health communication: A corpus linguistics approach (Corpus and Discourse) (Reprint ed.). London: Bloomsbury Academic.

Hasebe, Y., Lee, J., & Bekeš, A. (2019). *Readability measurement of Japanese texts based on levelled corpora. The Japanese language from an empirical perspective. Corpus-based studies and studies on discourse* (pp. 143–167). Japan: Sakura.

Hipgrave, D. (2011). Communicable disease control in China. *Journal of Global Health* 1(2), 224–238.

Hultman, T.G., & Westman, M. (1977). Gymnasistsvenska. Lund: Liber Laromedel.

Jacobi, C., van Atteveldt, W., & Welbers, K. (2015). Quantitative analysis of large amounts of journalistic texts using topic modelling. *Digital Journalism* 4(1), 89–106.

Jajosky, R.A., & Groseclose, S.L. (2004). Evaluation of reporting timeliness of public health surveillance systems for infectious diseases. *BMC Public Health* 4(29). https://doi.org/10.1186/1471-2458-4-29

Jelodar, H., Wang, Y., Yuan, C., Feng, X., Jiang, X., Li, Y., et al. (2018). Latent Dirichlet Allocation (LDA) and topic modeling: Models, applications, a survey. *Multimedia Tools and Applications* 78(11), 15169–15211.

Jensen, J.D. (2008). Scientific uncertainty in news coverage of cancer research: Effects of hedging on scientists and journalists credibility. *Human Communication Research* 34(3), 347–369.

Ji, M., Liu, Y., & Hao, T. (2021). Predicting health material accessibility: Development of machine learning algorithms. *JMIR Medical Informatics* 9(9), e29175.

Ji, M., & Sorensen, K. (2021). User-oriented healthcare translation. In Meng ji and Sara Laviosa (Editors), *Oxford handbook of translation and social practices* (pp. 1–23). Oxford: Oxford University Press.

Ji, M., Sorensen, K., & Bouillon, P. (2021). User-oriented healthcare translation and communication. In Meng Ji and Sara Laviosa (Eds.), *The Oxford handbook of translation and social practices* (pp. 1–23). New York: Oxford University Press.

Ji, M., Taibi, M., & Crezee, I. (2019). *Multicultural health translation, interpreting and communication.* Oxford and New York: Routledge.

Jian, L., , Xiang, H., & Le, G. (2022). English text readability measurement based on convolutional neural network: A hybrid network model. *Computational Intelligence and Neuroscience* 2022, 6984586.

Johnson, K. (2008). *Quantitative methods in linguistics.* Malden, MA: Blackwell Publishing.

Kandel, L., & Moles, A. (1958). Application de l'indice de Flesch à langue française. *Cahiers d'études de radio-télévision* 19, 253–279.

Kanungo, T., & Orr, D. (2009). Predicting the readability of short web summaries. WSDM, February 9–12, pp. 202–211. Barcelona, Spain.

Kanwal, J., Smith, K., Culbertson, J., & Kirby, S. (2017). Zipf's Law of Abbreviation and the Principle of Least Effort: Language users optimise a miniature lexicon for efficient communication. *Cognition* 165, 45–52.

Kasabwala, K., Agarwal, N., Hansberry, D.R., Baredes, S., & Eloy, J.A. (2012). Readability assessment of patient education materials from the American Academy of Otolaryngology – Head and Neck Surgery Foundation. *Otolaryngology–Head and Neck Surgery* 147(3), 466–471.

Kemper, S. (1983). Measuring the inference load of a text. *Journal of Educational Psychology* 75(3), 391–401.

Keselman, A., Logan, R., Smith, C.A., Leroy, G., & Zeng-Treitler, Q. (2008). Developing informatics tools and strategies for consumer-centered health communication. *Journal of the American Medical Informatics Association* 15(4), 473–483.

Kilgarriff, A., Husák, M., McAdam, K., Rundell, M., & Rychlý, P. (2008). Gdex: Automatically finding good dictionary examples in a corpus. In *Proceedings of the 13th EURALEX International Congress*, pp. 425–432. Barcelona, Spain.

Kim, J.H. (2009). Estimating classification error rate: Repeated cross-validation, repeated hold-out and bootstrap. *Computational Statistics & Data Analysis*, 53(11), 3735–3745.

Kim, S.J., & Fuemmeler, F. (2019). Detecting effective tobacco control messages via linguistic analysis and item response theory. *Cancer Epidemiology, Biomarkers, & Prevention* 28(3), 622.

Kincaid, J.P., Fishburne, R.P., Rogers, R.L., & Chissom, B.S. Derivation of new readability formulas (automated readability index, fog count and flesch reading ease formula) for navy enlisted personnel. *Institute for Simulation and Training, Research Report, 56.* (1975). http://stars.library.ucf.edu/istlibrary/56.

Kincaid, J., Fishburne, R., Rogers, R., & Chissom, L. (1975). Flesch-Kincaid Grade Level: *Technical report.* US Naval Air Station, Millington, TN.

King, H.R. (2019). Thinking about web accessibility. Morrisville, NC: Lulu Press.

Klare, G.R. (1963). The measurement of readability. Ames, Iowa: Iowa State University Press.

Kotani, K., Yoshimi, T., & Isahara, H. (2011). A machine learning approach to measurement of text readability for EFL learners using various linguistic features. *US-China Education Review B* 6, 767–777.

Kreuter, M.W., & McClure, S.M. (2004). The role of culture in health communication. *Annual Review of Public Health* 25(1), 439–455.

Kyne, D. L. (2020). Empirical evaluation of disaster preparedness for hurricanes in the Rio Grande Valley. *Progress in Disaster Science* 5, 100061. https://doi.org/10.1016/j.pdisas.2019.100061

Landsheere, G. (1963). Pour une application des tests de lisibilité de Flesch à la langue française. *Le travaile humaine* XXVI (–2), 141–154.

Larsson, P. (2006). *Classification into readability levels: Implementation and evaluation.* Master's thesis in computational linguistics, Dept. of Linguistics and Philology. Language Technology Programme. Uppsala University. 14 June.

Li, L. (2004). On the construction of the website of my country's local Center for Disease Control and Prevention. *Chinese Journal of Preventive Medicine* 5(1), 80–81.

Li, L.J., & Ge, G.C. (2009). Genre analysis: Structural and linguistic evolution of the English-medium medical research article (1985–2004). *English for Specific Purposes* 28(2), 93–104.

Lin, S. & Ji, M. (2019). Assessing linguistic comprehensibility of healthcare translation using the POCA model. In *Multicultural health translation, interpreting and communication.* London: Routledge.

Lin, X., Yang, F., Zhou, L., Yin, P., Kong, H., Xing, W., et al. (2012). A support vector machine-recursive feature elimination feature selection method based on artificial contrast variables and mutual information. *Journal of Chromatography B* 910, 149–155.

Lindell, M.K., & Perry, R.W. (2003). Communicating environmental risk in multiethnic communities (communicating effectively in multicultural contexts). London: Sage Publications.

Linsley, P., & Lawrence, M.J. (2007). Risk reporting by the largest UK companies: Readability and lack of obfuscation. Accounting, Auditing & Accountability Journal 20(4), 620–627.

Liu, Y., Ji, M., Shanshan Lin, S., Zhao, M., Lyv, Z. (2021). Combining readability formulas and machine learning for reader-oriented evaluation of online health resources. *IEEE Access* PP(99):1-1. https://doi.org/10.1109/ACCESS.2021.3077073

Loughran, T., & McDonald, B. (2014) Measuring readability in financial disclosures. *The Journal of Finance* 69(4), 1643–1671.

Lucisano, P., & Piemontese, M.E. (1988). Gulpease. Una formula per las predizione della difficultà dei testi in lingua italiana. *Scuola e Citta* 3, 57–68.

Lundgren, R., & McMakin, A. (2013). *Risk communication: A handbook for communicating environmental, safety, and health risks*, fourth edition. New York: Wiley. https://doi.org/10.1002/9781118645734

Lundgren, R.E., & McMakin, A.H. (2018). *Risk communication: A handbook for communicating environmental, safety, and health risks* (sixth edition). New York: Wiley-IEEE Press.

Maloney, S. (2005). Accessibility, nature, and quality of health information on the internet: A survey on osteoarthritis. *Rheumatology* 44(3), 382–385.

Mandic, C.G., Rudd, R., Hehir, T., & Acevedo-Garcia, D. (2010). Readability of special education procedural safeguards. *The Journal of Special Education* 45(4), 195–203.

Martinc, M., Pollak, S., Robnik-Šikonja, M. (2021). Supervised and unsupervised neural approaches to text readability. *Computational Linguistics* 47(1), 141–179.

Mastroianni, F., Chen, Y.C., Vellar, L., Cvejic, E., Smith, J.K., McCaffery, K.J., et al. (2019). Implementation of an organisation-wide health literacy approach to improve the understandability and actionability of patient information and education materials: A pre-post effectiveness study. *Patient Education and Counseling* 102(9), 1656–1661.

Matthiessen, C.M.I.M. (2013). Applying systemic functional linguistics in healthcare contexts. *Text & Talk*, 33(4–5), 437–466.

McCallum, D.B., Hammond, S.L., & Covello, V.T. (1991). Communicating about environmental risks: How the public uses and perceives information sources. *Health Education Quarterly* 18(3), 349–361.

McGraw, K.O., & Wong, S.P. (1992). A common language effect size statistic. *Psychological Bulletin* 111(2), 361–365.

McInnes, N., & Haglund, B.J.A. (2011). Readability of online health information: Implications for health literacy. *Informatics for Health and Social Care* 36(4), 173–189.

McLaughlin, G.H. (1969). SMOG grading: A new readability formula. *Journal of Reading* 222, 639–646.

Meillier, A., Patel, S., & Al-Osaimi, A.M.S. (2015). Readability of healthcare literature for hepatitis B and C. *Digestive Diseases and Sciences* 60(12), 3558–3562.

Mikolov, T., Karafiát, M., Burget, L., Černocký, J., & Khudanpur, S. (2010). Recurrent neural network-based language model. *11th Annual Conference of the International Speech Communication Association.*

Misra, P., Agarwal, N., Kasabwala, K., Hansberry, D.R., Setzen, M., & Eloy, J.A. (2012). Readability analysis of healthcare-oriented education resources from the American Academy of Facial Plastic and Reconstructive Surgery. *The Laryngoscope* 123(1), 90–96.

Murphy, B., Abdi, I., & Seale, H. (2020). Evaluating the health literacy demand and cultural appropriateness of online immunisation information available to refugee and migrant communities in Australia. *Vaccine* 38(41), 6410–6417.

Nadeem, F., & Ostendorf, M. (2018). Evaluating linguistic complexity for science texts. *Proceedings of the 13th Workshop on Innovative Use of NLP for Building Educational Applications*, pp. 45–55, New Orleans, Louisiana, 5 June.

Nasser, S.M.U., Cooke, G., Kranzer, K., Norris, S.L., Olliaro, P., & Ford, N. (2015). Strength of recommendations in WHO guidelines using GRADE was associated with uptake in national policy. *Journal of Clinical Epidemiology* 68(6), 703–707. https://doi.org/10.1016/j.jclinepi.2014.11.006

National Disaster Risk Information Services Capability. (2020). https://naturaldisaster.royalcommission.gov.au/system/files/2020-10/HAF.0012.0002.0003.pdf

Nepal, V., Banerjee, D., Perry, M., & Scott, D. (2012). Disaster preparedness of linguistically isolated populations. *Health Promotion Practice* 13(2), 265–271. http://www.jstor.org/stable/26739560

Nida, E. (1975). *Language structure and translation.* Stanford, CA: Stanford University Press.

Nivere, G., Camacho, V.M., Sia, S.R., Avilla, R., Butron, B., Fernandez, E.V., et al. (2017). Towards developing science of survival (SOS) pamphlets for typhoon, flashflood, storm surge and tsunami and for earthquakes and their aftermath: A pilot study. *International Electronic Journal of Environmental Education* 7(1), 59–77.

O'Brien, S., Federici, F., Cadwell, P., Marlowe, J., & Gerber, B. (2018). Language translation during disaster. *International Journal of Disaster Risk Reduction* 31, 627–636.

O'Hayre, J. and U.S. Department of the Interior, Bureau of Land Management (1966). *Gobbledygook Has Gotta Go.* Available at: https://books.google.com.au/books/about/Gobbledygook_Has_Gotta_Go.html?id=1yTeNg9bxGUC&redir_esc=y

Ogie, R.I., & Perez, P. (2020). Collaborative translation of emergency messages. *International Journal of Disaster Risk Reduction* 50, 101920. https://doi.org/10.1016/j.ijdrr.2020.101920

Pantula, M., & Kuppusamy, K.S. (2022). A machine learning-based model to evaluate readability and assess grade level for the web pages. *The Computer Journal* 64(4), 831–842.

Peter, M., McInnes-Dean, H., Fisher, J., Tapon, D., Chitty, L. S., & Hill, M. (2021). What's out there for parents? A systematic review of online information about prenatal microarray and exome sequencing. *Prenatal Diagnosis* 42(1), 97–108.

Peterson, S.E., & Ostendorf, M. (2009). A machine learning approach to reading level assessment. *Computer Speech and Language*, 23(1), 89–106.

Pianta, E., Bentivogli, L., & Girardi, C. (2002). MultiWordNet: Developing an aligned multilingual database. *First International Conference on Global WordNet*, pp. 292–302. Mysore, India.

Piantadosi, S.T., Tily, H., & Gibson, E. (2011). Word lengths are optimized for efficient communication. *Proceedings of the National Academy of Sciences* 108(9), 3526–3529.

Piantadosi, S.T. (2014). Zipf's word frequency law in natural language: A critical review and future directions. *Psychonomic Bulletin & Review* 21(5), 1112–1130.

Pilán, I., Volodina, E., & Johansson, R. (2014). Rule-based and machine learning approaches for second language sentence-level readability. *Proceedings of the Ninth Workshop on Innovative Use of NLP for Building Educational Applications*, pp. 174–184, Baltimore, Maryland, USA, June 26.

Prorok, J.C., Iserman, E.C., Wilczynski, N.L., & Haynes, R.B. (2012). The quality, breadth, and timeliness of content updating vary substantially for 10 online medical texts: An analytic survey. *Journal of Clinical Epidemiology* 65(12), 1289–1295.

Rayson, P. (2008). From key words to key semantic domains. *International Journal of Corpus Linguistics* 13(4), 519–549. https://doi.org/10.1075/ijcl.13.4.06ray

Rayson, P., Archer, D., Piao, S., & McEnery, A.M. (2004). The UCREL semantic analysis system. In *Proceedings of the beyond named entity recognition semantic labelling for NLP tasks workshop*, pp. 7–12. Lisbon.

Saarela, M., & Jauhiainen, S. (2021). Comparison of feature importance measures as explanations for classification models. *SN Applied Sciences* 3, 272.

Sbaffi, L., & Rowley, J. (2017). Trust and credibility in web-based health information: A review and agenda for future research. *Journal of Medical Internet Research* 19(6), e218.

Schwarm, S., & Ostendorf, M. (2005). Reading level assessment using support vector machines and statistical language models. In *Proceedings of the 43rd Annual Meeting of the Association for Computational Linguistics (ACL'05)*, pp. 523–530, Ann Arbor, Michigan. Association for Computational Linguistics.

Senter, R., & Smith, E.A. (1967). Automated readability index. Produced by Cincinnati University, Ohio. Available at: https://apps.dtic.mil/sti/citations/AD0667273

Shah, A.K., Yi, P.H., & Stein, A. (2015). Readability of orthopaedic oncology-related patient education materials available on the internet. *Journal of the American Academy of Orthopaedic Surgeons* 23(12), 783–788.

Shatilwe, J. T., Hlongwana, K., & Mashamba-Thompson, T. P. (2022). Pregnant adolescents and nurses perspectives on accessibility and utilization of maternal and child health information in Ohangwena Region, Namibia. *BMC Pregnancy and Childbirth* 22(1), 284. https://doi.org/10.1186/s12884-022-04619-w

Shedlosky-Shoemaker, R., Sturm, A.C., Saleem, M., & Kelly, K.M. (2008). Tools for assessing readability and quality of health-related web sites. *Journal of Genetic Counseling* 18(1), 49–59.

Sheehan, K. M., Flor, M., & Naplitano, D. (2013). A two-stage approach for generating unbiased estimates of text complexity. In *Proceedings of the Workshop on Natural Language Processing for Improving Textual Accessibility*, pp. 49–58. Association for Computational Linguistics.

Shoemaker, S.J., Wolf, M.S., & Brach, C. (2014). Development of the Patient Education Materials Assessment Tool (PEMAT): A new measure of understandability and actionability for print and audiovisual patient information. *Patient Education and Counseling* 96(3), 395–403.

Si, L., & Callan, J. (2001). A statistical model for scientific readability. *Proceedings of the 10th International Conference on Knowledge Management* (CIKM), pp. 574–576.

Škvorc, T., Krek, S., Pollak, S., & Arhad Holdt, S. (2018). Evaluation of statistical readability measures on Slovene texts. *Conference Jezikovne Technologije in Digitalna Humanistika*. Ljubljana, Slovenia.

Smith E.A., & Senter R.J. (1967). Automated Readability Index. *Armored Medical Research Laboratory (AMRL)*. Technical Report. 1–14.

Smith, E.A., & Kincaid, J.P. (1970). Derivation and validation of the automated readabiliy index for use with technical materials. *Human Factors* 12, 457–464.

Sørensen, K., & Brand, H. (2014). Health literacy lost in translations? *Health Promotion International* 29(4), 634–644.

Statista. (2024). Ranking of infectious diseases in China in 2019, by incidence. Available at: https://www.statista.com/statistics/861165/infectious-diseases-incidence-in-china/

Strekalova, Y.A., Krieger, J.L., Neil, J., Caughlin, J.P., Kleinheksel, A.J., & Kotranza, A. (2017). I understand how you feel: The language of empathy in virtual clinical training. *Journal of Language and Social Psychology* 36(1), 61–79.

Sung, Y-T., Chang, T-H, Lin, W-C, Hsieh, K-S, & Chang, K-E. (2016). Crie: An automated analyser for Chinese texts. *Behavior Research Methods*, 48(4), 1238–1251.

Szkody, E., & McKinney, C. (2021). Evaluating comforting messages with the sentiment analysis and social cognition engine. *Applied Psychology: Health and Well-Being* 14(2), 645–662.

Taylor-Clark, K., Koh, H., & Viswanath, K. (2007). Perceptions of environmental health risks and communication barriers among Low-SEP and racial/ethnic minority communities. *Journal of Health Care for the Poor and Underserved* 18 (4A), 165–183.

Thompson, T.L., & Harrington, N.G. (2021). *The Routledge handbook of health communication* (Routledge Communication Series) (3rd ed.). London: Routledge.

Todirascu, A., François, T., Bernhard, D., Gala, N., & Ligozat, A.L. (2016). Are cohesive features relevant for text readability evaluation. *COLING*, pp. 987–997, Osaka.

Toma, G., Guetterman, T.C., Yaqub, T., Talaat, N., & Fetters, M.D. (2017). A systematic approach for accurate translation of instruments: Experience with translating the Connor–Davidson Resilience Scale into Arabic. *Methodological Innovations* 10(3). https://doi.org/10.1177/2059799117741406

Tonelli, S., Tran Manh, K., & Pianta, E. (2012). Making readabiliy indices readable. In *Proceedings of the First Workshop on Predicting and Improving Text*

Readability for target reader populations, pp. 40–48. Montréal, Canada. Association for Computational Linguistics.

Uitdenbogerd, A.L. (2005). Readability of French as a foreign language and its uses. *Proceedings of the 10th Australasian Document Composing Symposium*, Sydney, Australia, 13 December.

Vajjala, S., & Lučić, I. (2018). OneStopEnglish corpus: Anew corpus for automatic readability assessment and text simplification. In *Proceedings of the Thirteenth Workshop on Innovative Use of NLP for Building Educational Applications*, pp. 297–304. New Orleans, Louisiana. Association for Computational Linguistics.

Vajjala, S., & Meurers, D. (2012). On improving the accuracy of readability classification using insights from second language acquisition. In *Proceedings of the 7th Workshop on Building Educational Applications Using NLP*, pp. 163–173. Montréal, Canada. Association for Computational Linguistics.

van Dijk, T.A., & Kintsch, W. (1983). *Strategies of discourse comprehension*. New York: Academic Press.

van Pelt, P.A., Drossaert, C.H.C., Kruize, A.A., Huisman, J., Radboud, J.E.M., Dolhain, N., & Wulffraat. (2015). Use and perceived relevance of health-related internet sites and online contact with peers among young people with juvenile idiopathic arthritis. *Rheumatology* 54(10), 1833–1841.

Varela-Centelles, P., Ledesma-Ludi, Y., Seoane-Romero, J., & Seoane, J. (2015). Information about oral cancer on the Internet: Our patients cannot understand it. *British Journal of Oral and Maxillofacial Surgery* 53(4), 393–395.

Vargha, A., & Delaney, H.D. (2000). A critique and improvement of the CL common language effect size statistics of McGraw and Wong. *Journal of Educational and Behavioral Statistics* 25(2), 101–132.

Venuti, L. (2017). *The translator's invisibility: a history of translation*. London: Routledge.

Verzani, J. (2005). *Using R for introductory statistics*. Boca Raton, FL: Chapman and Hall / CRC Press.

Villeneuve, M. et al. (2021). Applying a person-centred capability framework to inform targeted action on disability inclusive disaster risk reduction. *International Journal of Disaster Risk Reduction* 52, 101979. https://doi.org/10.1016/j.ijdrr.2020.101979

Visschers, V.H.M., Meertens, R.M., Passchier, W.W.F., & de Vries, N.N.K. (2009). Probability information in risk communication: A review of the research literature. *Risk Analysis* 29(2), 267–287.

Vold, E.T. (2006). Epistemic modality markers in research articles: A cross-linguistic and cross-disciplinary study. *International Journal of Applied Linguistics* 16(1), 61–87.

vor der Brück, T., & Hartrumpf, S. (2007). A semantically oriented readability checker for German. *Proceedings of the 3rd Language and Technology Conference*, pp. 270–274, Poznan, Poland, October.

vor der Brück, T., Hartfumpf, S., & Helbig, H. (2008). A readability checker with supervised learning using deep syntactic and semantic indicators. Proceedings of the 11th international multiconference: Information Society – IS 2008 – Language Technologies, Ljubljana, Slovenia, pp. 92–97.

Weinstein, N.D. (2000). Perceived probability, perceived severity, and health-protective behavior. *Health Psychology* 19(1), 65–74.

Whitney, J. (1997). Notes on methodology testing for differences with the non-parametric Mann Whitney U test. *Journal of Wound, Ostomy, and Continence Nursing* 24(1), 12–18.

Williams, A.R. Jr., Siegel, A., Burkett, J.R. (1974). Readability of textual material – a survey of the literature. Technical Training Division, Lowry Air Force Base, Colorado, 80230, July 1974. No. AFHRL-TR-74.

Wong, K., & Levi, J.R. (2016). Readability of paediatric otolaryngology information by children's hospitals and academic institutions. *The Laryngoscope* 127(4), E138–E144.

World Health Organization. (2020). Constitution of the World Health Organization, 49th edition. Available at: https://apps.who.int/gb/bd

World Health Organization. (2016). Evaluation of the impact of WHO publications: Evaluation brief – November 2016. Available at: https://cdn.who.int/media/docs/default-source/documents/evaluation/evaluation-brief-2016-impact-of-who-publication.pdf?sfvrsn=a49eef16_6&download=true

World Health Organization. (2025). Multilingualism and WHO. https://www.who.int/about/policies/multilingualism

World Health Organization. (1997). Process of translation and adaptation of instruments. Available at: https://www.who.int/substance_abuse/research_tools/translation/en/

World Health Organization. (2008). Toolkit on monitoring health systems strengthening. Health Information Systems. Available at: https://www.who.int/healthinfo/statistics/toolkit_hss/EN_PDF_Toolkit_HSS_InformationSystems.pdf

World Health Organization. World Health Organization eManual. VIII Information Products: EXECUTIVE BOARD EB123/7 123rd Session. Provisional agenda item 6.2.

World Health Organization. (2017). World Health Organization's Strategic Communications Framework for Effective Communications. https://www.who.int/docs/default-source/documents/communicating-for-health/communication-framework.pdf

Wu, L. (1999). Development and utilisation of WHO publications in China. *Health Informatics* 2, 36–38. http://www.aztsg.com/qikan/9173a4b5feb2ec2f1c18088b4ee468be.html

Xia, M., Kochmar, E., & Briscoe, T. (2016). Text readability assessment forsecond language learners. In *Proceedings of the 11th Workshop on Innovative Use of NLP for Building Educational Applications*, pp. 12–22. San Diego, CA. Association for Computational Linguistics.

Xiang, T., Gerber, B.J., & Zhang, F. (2018). Disaster management and the 'Whole Community' strategic approach: Assessing planning and preparedness efficacy for language access services. Midwest Political Science Association Conference, Chicago, Illinois, April 2018.

Xie, W., Ji, C., Hao, T., & Chow, C. (2021). Predicting the easiness and complexity of English health materials for international tertiary students with linguistically enhanced machine learning algorithms: Development and validation study. *JMIR Medical Informatics* 9(10), e25110. https://medinform.jmir.org/2021/10/e25110 and https://doi.org/10.2196/25110

Xie, W., Ji, M., Liu, Y., Hao, T., & Chow, C.Y. (2021). Predicting writing styles of online materials for children's health education using machine-learning assisted selection of semantic features (preprint). *JMIR Medical Informatics* 9(7), e30115. https://doi.org/10.2196/30115

Xie, J., & Liu, L. (2022). Identifying features of source and message that influence the retweeting of health information on social media during the COVID-19 pandemic. *BMC Public Health* 22, 805.

Xu, X. (1994). Control of communicable diseases in the People's Republic of China. *Asia Pacific Journal of Public Health* 7, 123–131.

Xu, W., Callison-Burch, C., & Napoles, C. (2015). problems in current text simplification research: New data can help. *Transactions of the Association for Computational Linguistics* 3, 283–297.

Yan, L., Xingtong, Z., Yidong, Z., Feng, M., Songjie, S., Yan, L., et al. (2021). Evaluation of the quality and readability of online information about breast cancer in China. *Patient Education and Counseling* 104(4), 858–864, https://doi.org/10.1016/j.pec.2020.09.012

Yancey, K., Pintard, A., & François, T. (2021). Investigating readability of French as a foreign language with deep learning and cognitive and pedagogical features. *Lingue e Linguaggio*, 2, 229–258.

Yaneva, V. (2016). *Assessing text and web accessibility for people with autism spectrum disorder*. Ph.D. thesis, University of Wolverhampton, 2016.

Yu-Ta, C., Yaw-Huei, C., & Yu-Chih, C. (2013). Assessing Chinese readability using term frequency and lexical chain. *Computational Linguistics and Chinese Language Processing* 18(2), 1–18.

Zamanian, M., & Heydari, P. (2012). Readability of texts: State of the art. *Theory and Practice in Language Studies* 2(1), 43–53.

Zhang, W., Yoshida, T., & Tang, X. (2008). Text classification based on multi-word with support vector machine. *Knowledge-Based Systems* 21(8), 879–886.

Zweig, M.H., & Campbell, G. (1993). Receiver-operating characteristic (ROC) plots: A fundamental evaluation tool in clinical medicine. *Clinical Chemistry* 39(4), 561–577.

Zwitter, A.V. (2014). Ugotavljanje avtorstva besedil: primer »Trenirkarjev«. In *zbornik Devete konference JezikoYne Tehnologije Informacijska dråba* ± IS, pp. 131–134.

Index

www.ingramcontent.com/pod-product-compliance
Lightning Source LLC
LaVergne TN
LVHW011813200926
848484LV00005B/1171
9781316512463